FROM THE AUTHOR OF "THE NO COMPROMISE BLACK SKIN CARE GUIDE" SERIES

MELANIN-RICH

ELEVATE YOUR UNDERSTANDING OF DARKER SKIN BY MASTERING ALL THINGS MELANIN

BY C. R. COOPER

The Skin Theologian

MELANIN-RICH

ELEVATE YOUR UNDERSTANDING OF DARKER SKIN BY MASTERING ALL THINGS MELANIN

BY C. R COOPER: THE SKIN THEOLOGIAN

IG: @theskintheologian

www.skintheologian.com
Let's Connect & Receive
Your FREE Pro Tip Guide

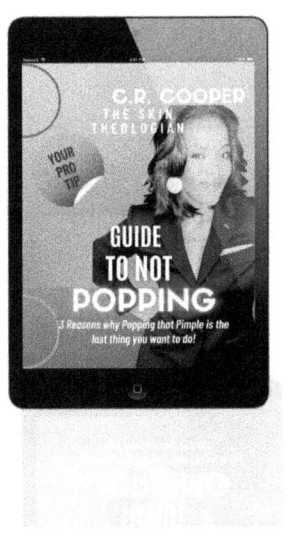

Cover and Science Diagrams
ILLUSTRATED BY SAM SINGH
www.samsinghillustration.com

© Copyright [C.R. Cooper: The Skin Theologian | Charmaine Cooper] [2024] - All rights reserved.

The content within this book may not be reproduced, duplicated or transmitted without direct written permission from the author or the publisher.

Under no circumstances will any blame or legal responsibility be held against the publisher, or author, for any damages, reparation, or monetary loss due to the information contained within this book. Either directly or indirectly. You are responsible for your own choices, actions, and results.

Legal Notice

This book is copyright-protected. This book is only for personal use. You cannot amend, distribute, sell, use, quote or paraphrase any part of the content within this book, without the consent of the author or publisher.

Disclaimer Notice

Please note the information contained within this document is for educational and entertainment purposes only. All effort has been expended to present accurate, up-to-date, and reliable, complete information. No warranties of any kind are declared or implied. Readers acknowledge that the author is not engaging in the rendering of legal, financial, medical or professional advice. The content within this book has been derived from various sources. Please consult a licensed professional before attempting any techniques outlined in this book.

By reading this document, the reader agrees that under no circumstances is the author responsible for any losses, direct or indirect, which are incurred as a result of the use of the information contained within this document, including, but not limited to, — errors, omissions, or inaccuracies.

CONTENTS

Introduction	13
Who Am I?	21
1. MELANIN-RICH: A GLOBAL EMBRACE	25
"We Are Far More Similar Than We Are Different"	26
Why Melanin-Rich?	27
How Do Clients Feel About the Term Melanin-Rich?	30
What Do Skin Professionals Think Of the Term Melanin-Rich?	31
Going Global	36
You Can't Say Anything Nowadays	37
What's Acceptable?	40
Communication That Counts	43
Skip These Outdated Terms	44
"Melanin-Rich": Should It Stay Or Go?	46
2. THE GRACE & TRUTH OF SKIN HEALTH EQUITY	51
Let's Talk Skin Health Equity	52
The Needle of Progress Is Moving	54
There's Still Work To Be Done	59
Why Sustainable Equity Is So Important	63
What's The Problem?	64
It's Time To Level-Up Training	67
Some Tech Has Improved but Challenges Still Remain	68

3. MELANIN-RICH AI: HOW AND WHY?   71
Me, Myself and AI   72
AI's Precision in Understanding Melanin-Rich Skin   74
AI's Role in Mitigating Bias and Fostering Inclusivity   75
AI and Skin Education   80
Opportunities for AI to Support CQ   82
Emerging Tech and Future Trends   82

4. MELANOCYTES: THE GOOD | THE BAD | THE SCIENCE   85
What is Melanin?   86
Unriddling the Melanocyte   88
The Building Blocks of Melanocytes   89
Understanding Constitutive and Facultative Color   97

5. STEP INTO THE (MELANIN-RICH) CLASSROOM   113
Why CQ Ed is Key   114
Melanin-Rich: Fundamentals   119
Melanin-Rich: Intermediary   125
Melanin-Rich: Advanced Level   134

6. MELANIN-RICH: PRO PERSPECTIVES   139
A Skin Pro's Perspective   140

7. LET'S GET CLINICAL   161
The Science Behind Skin   162
Genetics and Melanin   163

8. STEP INTO THE TREATMENT ROOM   171
Understanding Your Clientele   172
Setting the Scene   173
The Research Phase   174
Get The Booking   177
The First Appointment   178

9. OFF LIMITS: MELANIN-RICH INFLAMMATORY DISEASES, DISORDERS AND TREATMENT BOUNDARIES ... 183
What Does The Industry Look Like Today? ... 184
Dermatologists Represent! ... 185
Primary Skin Disorders Skin Pros Should Know ... 191
Skincare and Beauty Industry ... 197
Academic Publications and Resources ... 201
Real Improvement to Industry Inclusion and Diversity ... 204
Medi-Aesthetic Collaborations Serve Melanin-Rich Clients ... 205
The 3-Tip Professional Guide to Client Care ... 209
Lead with Humanity ... 209

Conclusion ... 215
Glossary of Resources and Terms ... 217
Notes ... 231

INTRODUCTION

MELANIN-RICH SKIN IS NOT COMPLICATED.

All skin is more similar than it is different.

There, I said it.

You might think that's a weird statement to open up within a book dedicated to understanding Melanin-Rich skin.

The truth is that when it comes to our skin, we all have a lot more in common than we think. Humanity is a beautiful race, and almost every person in the world has melanin in their skin.

To be able to celebrate our differences and experiences, it's important that we first celebrate what binds us together. And one of those things is our beautiful skin.

The things we have in common help us to understand our uniqueness so that everyone can be represented with unapologetic awareness.

This is where Melanin-Rich skin comes in. Melanin-Rich skin hasn't had enough curriculum, education or attention in decades - never mind content, reference points and documented experiences. Other skin tones have had far more representation and awareness, even though more people across the world have Melanin-Rich skin.

Thankfully, things are starting to improve (slowly), but things still need to move forward. We need to pick up the pace ASAP.

You may be familiar with The No Compromise Black Skin Care Guide Series, which might be why you're now reading this book. This is the educational, yet conversational, book series I wrote for Skin Pros, consumers and those looking to enhance their knowledge.

And people *are* looking for that knowledge and understanding of Melanin-Rich skin, believe me. I've connected with international professionals who are looking for support in enhancing their awareness of working with Melanin-Rich skin.

I've presented to rooms filled with people from all different backgrounds, brands and experiences with one common thread between them - *they want to know more.*

I'd love to invite you to take a deep breath and brace yourself as we delve into the riveting exploration of Melanin-Rich skin. This isn't your typical stroll through the pages, but don't rush through either. I'd like you to explore the nuanced world of Melanin-Rich skin one bit at a time. No matter what you may or may not know already about Melanin-Rich skin, I hope this book brings you beyond physiology, socio-economics, and science. It's a narrative that celebrates the profound humanity embedded in understanding the brilliance of Melanin-Rich skin.

As much as I'm talking about a lack of awareness of working with and understanding Melanin-Rich skin, recently it feels like melanin's become something of a buzzword.

MELANIN-POPPIN', MELANIN-GLOW, MELANATED are phrases you'll see all over social media and in editorials. But actual MELANIN is way more than a trendy, cute colloquialism that's used for likes and relatability.

Melanin has a scientific origin. One that allows us great insight and understanding into how to care for melanin-related concerns and the cells that produce it.

These cells are called melanocytes and need to be at the heart of understanding Melanin-Rich skin. So let's get into it in this book.

It's an exploration of Melanin-Rich skin. And the journey we need to be on to have a greater understanding of the cultural, educational and resource basis when it comes to understanding it.

A Snapshot of the Melanin-Rich Beauty Space

Let's take an overview of where we're at when it comes to Melanin-Rich skincare.

The good, the bad, the progress and where the industry needs to pick up the pace.

- There are more Black-owned brands and diverse, inclusive brands that cater to every skin type and tone. Brands like Fenty Beauty, Black Girl Sunscreen and Pat McGrath have founders who have created brands based on their lived experiences.
- Google has launched the Monk Skin Tone Scale[1] as an alternative scale more inclusive than other industry standards.

- Black beauty brand incubators, such as the BrainTrust Founders Studio, and formulators, such as Sula Labs, have risen to create beauty products from the experience and knowledge points of someone with Melanin-Rich skin.
- Vogue Business[2] named 'Melanin-Rich skin care' as beauty's next business opportunity at the end of 2022, and called it a category that's long overdue for significant investment.
- "Melanin-Safe" skincare is rising in popularity[3] - products that have been formulated and created with Skin of Color in mind.
- Initiatives like the Fifteen Percent Pledge have been implemented to save 15 percent of dedicated shelf space to Black-owned brands at major retailers like Nordstrom, Macy's, Sephora and Ulta. This is up from less than 3 percent for many of them.[4]
- Black households above the median US income continue to enter the beauty market, buying luxury skincare, cosmetics and treatments. As a group, Black Americans are increasing their spending on beauty products slightly faster than the total US market. Black consumers spent $8 billion on beauty and black cosmetics – a 10% increase compared to the total market's 9% growth.[5]

- More than 11% of all beauty customers are Black—and yet Black brands account for a mere 2.5% of total beauty industry revenues.[6]
- Research by McKinsey[7] had some disappointing findings regarding Black consumers and beauty retail, including:
- Black consumers are three times more likely to be dissatisfied than non-Black consumers with their options for hair care, skincare and makeup.
- Black customers regularly experience a lack of knowledge from sales associates. This might be something that surprises you - but it doesn't honestly surprise me. In my experience, the main reason for this is a lack of confidence, training and experience from Skin Pros and a lack of diversity in equipment device technology.
- Black consumers aren't offered the right products or professional services to meet their needs.
- Black-owned brands make up less than 7% of what's on the shelves.

It's a mixed bag of wins, losses and "do better" across the board. But even with these disappointments, there's a whole lot of progress in there, and I'm here for it.

SKIN THEOLOGIAN'S SKINSIGHT

Want a deeper understanding of some key skincare terms you need to know especially regarding Melanin-Rich skin?

Hit the glossary section at the end of this book for a more-than-skin-deep definition of terms, ingredients and resources you need to know when it comes to Skin Health Equity.

You're welcome.

WHO AM I?

C.R. COOPER - SKIN THEOLOGIAN

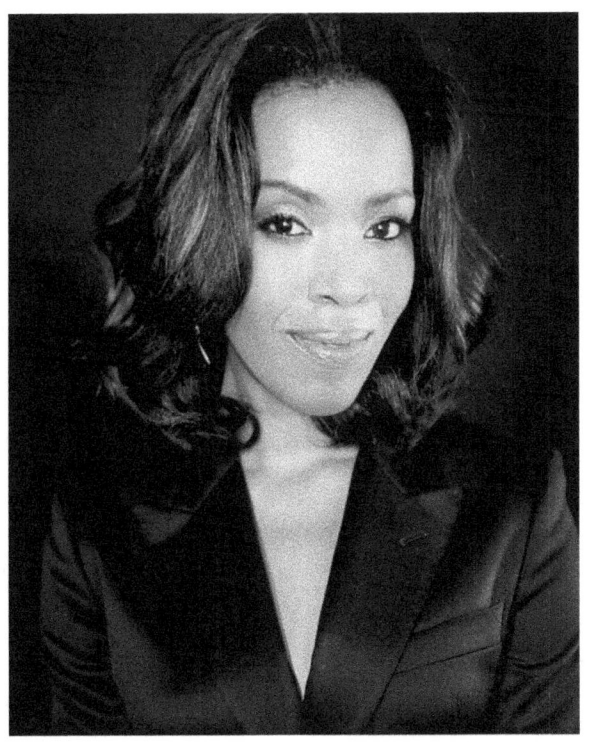

I'm C.R. Cooper, your Skin Theologian. Many, call me Char.

Ever wonder who's behind the scenes challenging the norms in Skin Health Equity education? That would be me.

With almost 28 years in the industry (at the time of publication), I've worn various hats - from Education Manager to jet-setting Master Educator for a global Skin Institute.

My journey has taken me across borders, educating on skin health practices and collaborating with companies & clients to achieve skin health goals to be proud of. Picture this: standing in front of Skin Pros worldwide, passionately advocating for Skin Health Equity, Cultural Intelligence (CQ), and a universal standard of skin health education that embraces every skin type, especially the most underrepresented skin - Melanin-Rich skin.

Maybe you've come across my brainchild, The No Compromise Black Skin Care Guide series, a trilogy sparked in 2020, first released in 2021 with a simple hope — to move the needle on Skin Health Equity. Fast forward a few years, and the ripple effect has been incredible. The advocacy has grown, and the movement is thriving.

But here's the tea – while culturally sensitive and diverse skin health practices should be the norm, your average client often finds themselves navigating the beauty landscape without adequate support. And Skin Professionals? Some are overwhelmed, even stressed, when faced with treating unfamiliar skin types, be it any age, gender, or the myriad shades of Melanin-Rich skin.

Confidence levels are a concern, and rightly so. Properly understanding Melanin-Rich skin is an ongoing challenge. I've engaged with Skin Professionals worldwide over the years, witnessing the growing educational need. Clients who have Melanin-Rich skin, frustrated or even fearful of approaching new businesses due to a lack of support, are seeking understanding. And our new Skin Pros? They're stressed about the unknown.

But here's where I come in. As a Skin Pro and Educator, I'm here to change the narrative. I firmly believe that every Skin Professional has the right to be competent in treating all skin, especially Melanin-Rich skin, which, by the way, spans beyond just Black skin. It's about understanding the physiological intricacies that make each skin similar, yet unique.

The call for Skin Health Equity practices resonates globally. I've been on the ground, listening to concerns from Clinic and Spa owners, Skin Professional students, graduates, and clients across countries.

Having been recognized with the Aestheticians Choice Awards 2024 for Favorite Contributing Writer by Dermascope, I take education seriously. Contributing to Professional Trade Magazines like Australia's Professional Beauty, Global Dermascope, and Pema Journal has been an honor, amplifying the voice of Skin Health Equity.

The journey continues, and the need for equity in all aspects of Skin Health, especially for Melanin-Rich skin, is ever-growing. This task isn't for a lone author or a single company. It's a collective effort, a chorus of voices from Skin Professionals, Educators, organizations and companies, all contributing to lasting change.

So, let's embark on this journey together, embracing real 'Skin-fluence' and making waves of positive change in the world of skincare.

1

MELANIN-RICH: A GLOBAL EMBRACE

This term has emerged in response to a growing societal awareness...

In this chapter, you'll explore:

- What "Melanin-Rich" actually means and whether it's here to stay
- The importance of communication with your clients
- The terms that it's time to press pause on

"WE ARE FAR MORE SIMILAR THAN WE ARE DIFFERENT"

Skin is skin. I know this book is a resource for Melanin-Rich skin, but realistically most skin tones and structures have similar basic needs.

However, confusion or a lack of comfort when working with skin that's significantly different from our own can lead to an over-cautious approach that leaves clients feeling misunderstood.

I understand. It's what you're familiar with - or unfamiliar with. Depending on where you are in the world, the education you received and the hands-on, lived experience that you've had with clients will mean that you will have had a life as a Skin Professional that's unique to you. That's wonderful and is one of the reasons why I love the industry so much. It's diverse and has people from all walks of life.

However, we don't always know who's going to walk through the door of our skin space, so getting educated and understanding all skin types and tones is an essential part of being a successful Skin Pro.

That's why this educational resource around Melanin-Rich skin exists. Let's take it back to basics so we all understand where we're at.

WHY MELANIN-RICH?

I'd recommend using the term Melanin-Rich. It's positive, it acknowledges a client's skin and it shows your understanding as a Skin Professional.

Melanin-Rich skin refers to skin that has higher levels of melanin, the pigment responsible for its color. This type of skin is commonly found in individuals with diverse backgrounds, particularly those with ancestry from regions with intense sunlight, like Africa, Asia, and some parts of the Middle East and Latin America. Melanin-Rich skin comes in various shades.

It's an inclusive term that celebrates darker skin tones without running the risk of misunderstanding someone's heritage. It acknowledges their skin, and why it's something to be proud of, without making detailed assumptions. That's why we're using it here.

All skin types and tones are beautiful, so it's important that we refer to them inclusively and with love. Just like with the term "Melanin-Rich skin".

It avoids confusion and avoids making clients feel uncomfortable or misunderstood by the person who's working with their precious skin.

The term "Melanin-Rich" has gained acceptance and popularity because it focuses on celebrating the diversity and beauty of various skin tones without attaching negative connotations or stereotypes.

Unlike outdated terms that often carry historical baggage, medical terminology or perpetuated racial biases, "Melanin-Rich" emphasizes the abundance of melanin pigment positively and inclusively. It doesn't pigeonhole individuals into restrictive categories but acknowledges the richness and uniqueness of diverse skin tones.

This term has emerged in response to a growing societal awareness and appreciation for diversity, promoting inclusivity and respect for various ethnic backgrounds. It serves as a way to recognize and celebrate the presence of melanin across different skin tones, from darker to lighter shades, without marginalizing or categorizing individuals solely based on their appearance.

"Melanin-Rich" also aligns with efforts toward cultural intelligence and inclusivity in various fields, including skincare, beauty, and healthcare. It acknowledges the importance of melanin in protecting against sun damage and reflects a shift towards a more comprehensive and respectful language that appreciates the wide spectrum of skin tones found across different ethnicities and cultures.

Ultimately, it's a term that embraces diversity, promoting a positive and empowering narrative around skin color and ethnicity. For those of you who know my work on Cultural Intelligence (CQ) within the skin space, you'll know exactly why this term has my CQ stamp of approval.

SKIN THEOLOGIAN'S SKINSIGHT

According to Google Trends,[1] searches for "Melanin Rich" have more than tripled globally over the last 5 years, showing that it's being adopted and used more widely across the globe.

The term #melaninrich[2] has also been used on 757,000 Instagram posts on the leading image-sharing platform at the time of this publication.

As a hashtag, #melaninrich[3] has also had 6.2 million views on the short-form video-sharing site TikTok - something that's important when it comes to the beauty industry trends cycle, as well as cultural change, right now.

It's entered the global discourse and it looks like people are continuing to identify and resonate with it.

HOW DO CLIENTS FEEL ABOUT THE TERM MELANIN-RICH?

Opinions among individuals with higher levels of melanin regarding the term "Melanin-Rich" can vary. For many, the term represents a positive shift in language, acknowledging and celebrating the beauty and diversity of skin tones. It's seen as a way to embrace and affirm the presence of melanin in various ethnicities, fostering pride in one's natural skin color.

Some individuals appreciate the term "Melanin-Rich" as it moves away from outdated or derogatory terms, providing a more inclusive and respectful way to describe diverse skin tones. It promotes a sense of unity and empowerment within communities that have historically faced discrimination or negative stereotypes based on their skin color.

However, it's essential to recognize that opinions can differ among individuals. While many embrace the term "Melanin-Rich," others might prefer different descriptors or feel that it oversimplifies the complexity of skin diversity within various ethnic groups.

Some individuals may prefer to be identified by their specific cultural or ethnic backgrounds rather than a term focused solely on melanin. It's ok if they feel like that, and it's ok to be respectful of it - just establish it with them in your communication with the client.

WHAT DO SKIN PROFESSIONALS THINK OF THE TERM MELANIN-RICH?

Skincare professionals generally view the term "Melanin-Rich" positively as it highlights the importance of melanin in skin health.

Many professionals appreciate this term for its inclusivity and accuracy in describing the skin's pigmentation levels, acknowledging the role of melanin in various skin types. It also takes any ambiguity around how they should be having conversations with their clients and shows that they have an understanding of their needs.

For skincare professionals, understanding and recognizing melanin levels are crucial aspects of providing effective and personalized skincare solutions.

The term "Melanin-Rich" helps professionals acknowledge the unique characteristics and needs of different skin tones. It allows them to tailor treatments, SPF recommendations and skincare regimens specifically to address the protective and maintenance needs of higher melanin levels, promoting healthy and radiant skin.

The term aligns with the efforts of Skin Pros to promote diversity and inclusivity within the industry. It helps foster a more comprehensive understanding of skin tones, encouraging professionals to embrace cultural intelligence and provide respectful and tailored skincare advice to clients from diverse ethnic backgrounds.

SKIN THEOLOGIAN'S SKINSIGHT

I asked my international network of Skin Pros what they thought of the term "Melanin-Rich skin", for both clients and professionals.

Here's what they had to say:

• Absolutely love the term! I feel like most don't know/feel intimidated by the word and how to address deeper skin tones. Either they don't have a large client base of clients with deeper skin tones or haven't had enough practice. I feel like it's also a word thrown around a lot by companies or businesses.

• I wonder if some people who are not melanin-rich feel slightly insulted? As a Skin Pro with experience with all ethnicities, do others without Melanin-Rich skin feel like they'd be melanin-poor? I don't want any of my clients to feel bad. How else could it be worded? Not sure.

• I think that the term is used more now and has been accepted more in the industry.

• I personally feel as though "Melanin-Rich skin" appropriately captures a wide range of skin tones while using respectful and professional terminology that clients can actually understand.

• Melanin-Rich skin stands out for inclusivity. It's well-received by Skincare Pros and clients.

• I think it's good. I'm always thinking about the science of the skin and I don't think clients consider the depth of complexity when it comes to treating different levels of melanin.

• In the industry, the term is understood and it's all-encompassing for all skin tones. But to clients, more education is still needed. It's a complex term.

• I think this is a very classy way to refer to Women of color.

It's empowering and creates a heightened awareness of our skin's specific care and its needs. It creates a sense of unity from lighter shades to the deeper ones.

- Melanin-Rich skin doesn't have the space to sit in the industry as much as other terms, in my opinion.

- Melanin-Rich is an elevated term that is relevant to both Skin Professionals and consumers.

- Melanin-Rich is absolutely beautifully put.

- I personally feel fine with it, but I am not positive it sits well with the larger community. I feel that the term skin of color is more acceptable/palatable and makes people feel more comfortable.

- I love the term Melanin-Rich, I think it's more inclusive, feels more personal and sweet.

- I think the term sits very well in our industry, we just need more of us using the term!

- The term Melanin-Rich skin describes the beauty of our skin.

- I genuinely think it's perfection and couldn't think of a more appropriate beautiful word to describe our clients with darker skin tones. In fact, I use this word in my salon ALL the time.

- I have found the term to fit seamlessly into a conversation with Skin Pros, students and clients with Melanin-Rich skin. It feels natural to say.

- Melanin-Rich skin is the perfect term to use because it immediately eliminates division.

- Melanin-Rich is something I fully embraced, fostering inclusivity among Skin Pros & clients, surpassing other industry terms.

- I always get funny looks from my patients when I use that term in the UK. Like I'm offending them.

- It promotes inclusivity and is a positive term everyone can use referring to Fitzpatrick 4, 5 & 6.

- The term is embraced positively, but awareness is needed to avoid tokenism. Diversity in products and training is crucial.

As you can see, there is a real variety of perspectives in there, though it's overwhelmingly positive feedback for the term. The Skin Pros I asked represented a real mix of experience, client base and world locations, so I expected that would be the case.

GOING GLOBAL

We have to remember that melanin is relevant across a diverse range of skin types and ethnicities. It isn't just used to refer to Black skin.

In our globalized society, the spectrum of melanin expands all over the world to people with heritage from everywhere: Hispanic, Mediterranean, South East Asian, Asian, Caribbean and mixed backgrounds.

Across these diverse backgrounds, melanin plays a pivotal role in protecting the skin from the sun's harmful UV rays. While individuals from these ethnicities may have varying levels of melanin, its presence is essential for shielding the skin from some levels of UV-induced damage.

Not all Melanin-Rich skin looks the same. It runs a spectrum of shades and tones, which means that assumptions don't cut it. Someone could have a lighter complexion but still have a heritage that's rich in melanin.

As I've mentioned before, all shades of skin contain melanin. It's relevant for everyone, but especially for skin that is Melanin-Rich.

Understanding and appreciating melanin's role across a global array of skin types is so important for promoting comprehensive skincare practices and UV daylight protection across diverse ethnicities and cultures.

YOU CAN'T SAY ANYTHING NOWADAYS

I've heard people express their concerns about not knowing the right thing to say, or how to talk about Melanin-Rich skin without causing offense or upset.

"You can't say anything nowadays without someone getting upset!"

"The terms change all the time and I never know what's right to say!"

"I find it just easier not to refer to it at all so no one's offended."

Do any of those statements sound familiar? I've heard all of these concerns and more. They're rooted in a good place deep down - the desire not to cause upset, offense or hurt to another person, which is always positive - but by choosing not to address it or educate themselves Skin Pros are kind of doing everyone a disservice.

By sitting in that place of ignorance and not taking the time to understand skin that is Melanin-Rich, Skin Professionals run the risk of:

- Alienating their clients with Melanin-Rich skin
- Carrying out treatments without a full understanding of the skin they're working on
- Delivering poor client consultations
- Having ineffective communication with their clients
- Not bringing inclusive practices into their treatment space
- Missing an opportunity for development and education
- Getting left behind

See how important it is to get comfortable in talking about all shades and tones of skin? It's essential for the professional-to-client relationship.

And it doesn't need to be complicated, worrying or cause for alarm. Melanin-Rich skin is complex, not complicated. Understanding this difference is key.

SKIN THEOLOGIAN'S SKINSIGHT

One thing I've seen before is Skin Professionals that don't understand that their lens or perspective may be problematic, as others don't have the same experiences or knowledge.

For example, a Caucasian Skin Professional may refer to a Black client as being "dark-skinned". Black skin comes in lots of different shades and the term "dark-skinned" can have different connotations within different communities.

While that client may be "dark-skinned" compared to someone with Caucasian skin, within their own community they may not be considered "dark" at all.

That's why it's so important to have an awareness of communities other than your own, and not just base relevance on a comparison to yourself.

Even widely-accepted terms like "people of color" can be a challenge as they're used to "othering" those with Melanin-Rich skin in comparison to Caucasian skin tones.

WHAT'S ACCEPTABLE?

Language and culture are fluid. Always has been, always will be. What was the done thing and acceptable practice 50, 15, 5 years ago is constantly evolving, changing and growing.

I'm not completely unsympathetic when people say they're not sure what to say. As I mentioned earlier, it comes from a place of concern rather than malice. But that doesn't mean you shouldn't get up to date in a hurry.

Skin Pros might use various respectful and inclusive terms when referring to individuals with higher levels of melanin in their skin. Here are a few appropriate terms:

- **Melanin-Rich skin** - this term celebrates the abundance of melanin, acknowledging the diversity and beauty of darker skin tones without making assumptions about heritage.
- **Darker skin tones** - describes skin with higher melanin levels respectfully and inclusively. It's factual. These skin tones are darker when it comes to skin tone categorization (such as the Fitzpatrick Scale or Google's Monk Skin Tone Scale).

- **Deeper skin shade** - this is used in a similar context to darker skin tones and means the same thing.
- **Richly pigmented skin** - indicates skin with a higher concentration of pigmentation, highlighting its beauty and natural diversity.
- **Melanated skin** - This is a unique one as it usually refers to skin with higher levels of melanin, basically in the same way as "Melanin-Rich". But for accuracy, this is incorrect. Professionally, all skin tones are Melanated. We will get to the science of this later in the book, but Melanated does not exclusively describe skin that is Melanin-Rich - it describes all degrees of melanin.
- **Skin of color** - this term is commonly used as a catch-all for skin that's in the Melanin-Rich category. It's widely used and may be understood more easily by clients.

If you know what someone's heritage is (and by know, I mean KNOW) then by all means, you can refer to them as that. This could be Black, Hispanic, Latina, South East Asian, Asian etc. But really, only if you know. Please don't just try and guess, and hope for the best.

Having this awareness shows you've taken the time to get to know them and their skin and it won't be a spoiler to them - they know what their heritage is too.

Ultimately, if in doubt I'd recommend using Melanin-Rich. It's positive, it acknowledges a client's skin and it shows your understanding as a Skin Professional.

It's essential to use terms that show appreciation for diversity, avoid stereotypes, and prioritize inclusivity when discussing or addressing individuals with higher melanin levels in their skin. Respecting the preferences of the individual is crucial when choosing terminologies in professional settings. It's one of the signature criteria for holding a CQ conversation with clients.

Something else to keep in mind, while asking your clients what they prefer is acceptable, you shouldn't leave it down to your clients to "correct you if they feel so strongly about it" (I've heard this too).

It can be tiring and triggering dealing with microaggressions or correcting people all day long about what they should and shouldn't say. Some clients may not feel comfortable starting that conversation on a negative foundation (but believe me, some *will* and it'll affect that important relationship you have with them). Some clients will just shut down and you won't ever see them again.

FYI, a microaggression is a subtle, often unintentional, comment or action that communicates derogatory or negative messages, reflecting underlying biases or stereotypes about a person's race, gender or other aspects of their identity.

Communication is key in any client relationship, and that's no different when it comes to talking about skin tone.

COMMUNICATION THAT COUNTS

As a Skin Pro, effective communication with clients - whatever their skin type, tone, age or needs - is vital for several reasons: fostering trust, understanding and ensuring optimal care.

When clients feel heard and understood, it builds a stronger rapport, making them more likely to follow professional advice and treatment plans. Trust is key when it comes to that all-important client-professional relationship, encouraging clients to return for continued care.

Plus it makes the client's experience better, and your working day runs way smoother.

Building trust begins with open communication, allowing clients to openly share their concerns, preferences, and aspirations for their skincare journey. When clients feel truly heard and understood, it creates a stronger bond, increasing their likelihood of following professional advice and treatment plans. Trust forms the bedrock of this relationship.

Moreover, inclusive communication empowers Skin Professionals to fully grasp the unique needs of each client. By actively listening to their concerns, lifestyle factors, and medical history, Skin Pros gain valuable insights into individual skin conditions and goals. This information becomes the cornerstone for crafting personalized treatment plans that precisely target specific concerns and desired outcomes, ensuring tailored and effective skincare solutions.

Clear communication isn't just about dialogue—it's also about educating clients. Skin Pros can explain skincare routines, products, and procedures in a way that's understandable and suitable for each client's skin. This empowerment enables informed decision-making, encouraging clients to adhere to prescribed routines and dispelling misconceptions about proper skin care practices for long-term skin health.

SKIP THESE OUTDATED TERMS

As I mentioned earlier, language and culture are fluid - I think that's great as it shows we're always developing, growing and moving forward to become more inclusive.

However, I get that this is why people get confused or uncomfortable about what to say - especially older generations who may have seen different terms for similar things fall in and out of acceptability. But we can all adapt and learn, at any age.

Let's run through some outdated terms for Melanin-Rich skin, so you can skip them in your conversations with clients about their skin.

- **Colored** - historically used to describe individuals with darker skin tones, but considered outdated and carrying negative connotations due to its historical use during times of racial segregation. I'll acknowledge that this is still used in some parts of the world, such as South Africa, without offense. But it's best to skip it entirely.
- **Olive-skinned** - while not inherently offensive, this term has been associated with categorizing Mediterranean or Hispanic individuals based

on skin color, sometimes oversimplifying or stereotyping diverse skin tones.
- **Ethnic minority** - while not directly related to skin tone, the term "ethnic minority" has been used in the past to describe individuals with darker skin tones, but it can be seen as outdated or limiting in representing the diverse backgrounds and experiences within these groups.

It's essential to use respectful and inclusive language that celebrates diversity and avoids stereotypes or outdated terms when referring to skin tones and origins.

These terms will all probably change in the future, and it's on us to stay aware and up to date with that.

"MELANIN-RICH": SHOULD IT STAY OR GO?

While none of us can predict the future as accurately as I'm sure we'd all like to, there are signs that the term "Melanin-Rich" has some longevity yet.

Not all parts of the world, or all Skin Pros resonate with the term Melanin-Rich, as you saw in the earlier feedback. The truth is, we don't know what the future of our space will look like. This isn't necessarily a campaign for the best terminology as much as it is a quest for a respectful understanding of the nuances of skin that has been overlooked for many years. Ultimately, use terms that feel right for you and your clients.

The term "Melanin-Rich" appears to be here to stay due to several important factors shaping its acceptance and longevity in contemporary language and cultural discourse. Here's what I think may be contributing to this:

- The term embodies a movement towards inclusivity and empowerment. It celebrates the beauty and diversity of skin tones, promoting a positive narrative that embraces everyone without marginalization or stereotypes.
- There's a growing societal awareness and appreciation for diversity and representation across various platforms, from beauty and fashion to healthcare and social activism. The term "Melanin-Rich" reflects this cultural shift, acknowledging the importance of melanin in skin health across different ethnicities and cultures.
- Within the skincare and health industries, there's a heightened understanding of the significance of melanin in protecting against

sun damage and skin-related conditions. As Skin Professionals emphasize tailored skincare regimens for diverse skin tones, the term "Melanin-Rich" becomes an essential descriptor for addressing specific skin needs.

- The term has received a generally positive reception from diverse communities, especially those historically marginalized or misrepresented based on their skin tones. Its widespread acceptance signifies a shift towards more respectful and inclusive language, emphasizing pride and appreciation for one's natural skin color.
- As society continues to evolve, conversations around race, ethnicity, and diversity remain significant. Terms like "Melanin-Rich" contribute to these ongoing discussions, driving home the importance of understanding and appreciating the diverse spectrum of skin tones present across global populations. They're bringing things together rather than separating them.

As I also mentioned earlier, the term Melanin-Rich continues to grow in searches year after year, showing that it's staying relevant and used by people when they're seeking information online - usually a good indicator of how people are feeling and behaving about something.

Given these factors and the term's positive reception across various sectors, it seems likely that "Melanin-Rich" will continue as a respectful and inclusive way to talk to your clients, contributing to a broader conversation about diversity, representation, and cultural appreciation. I'm a fan and I hope it sticks around longer.

2

THE GRACE & TRUTH OF SKIN HEALTH EQUITY

It's also about money.

There, I said it.

In this chapter, you'll discover:

- What Skin Health Equity is
- Why sustainable equity is an important consideration
- Where there are progress and challenges in Skin Health Equity

LET'S TALK SKIN HEALTH EQUITY

If you've read any of my previous work, or you follow me on any of my platforms then hopefully you're already familiar with skin health equity. I talk about it a lot - and with good reason!

For the uninitiated (don't worry, by the end of this book we'll have you all over Skin Health Equity!), let's start with the basics of the term first.

Skin Health Equity is about ensuring fairness, impartiality and equality in the access to skincare resources, treatments and information across diverse populations.

It aims to emphasize and eliminate disparities and barriers that prevent individuals from all ethnicities, cultural backgrounds or socioeconomic statuses from receiving adequate and appropriate skincare and dermatological care.

This concept recognizes that various factors, including race, ethnicity, geographical location, economic status, and cultural practices, can significantly impact an individual's access to skincare resources and healthcare services. Skin Health Equity seeks to address these disparities by promoting equal opportunities for all individuals to achieve optimal skin health, regardless of their background.

Unfortunately, this hasn't always been the case. Research[1] has shown that dermatology textbooks only contain between 4 and 18% darker skin tones. This means that many medical practitioners are unaware of how skin conditions manifest on all skin shades - this leads to issues with diagnosis and treatment. It wasn't being taught, and people weren't learning.

Achieving Skin Health Equity involves several key aspects, such as providing accessible and affordable skincare products, offering culturally competent care, professional devices for Melanin-Rich skin and education, ensuring representation in research and clinical trials, advocating for policies that support diversity and inclusivity in skincare, and empowering communities to prioritize skin health.

Skin Health Equity aims to create a level playing field where everyone has the same opportunities and access to high-quality skincare resources, education, treatments, modalities and information, irrespective of their cultural, racial or socioeconomic differences. It's about ensuring fairness and inclusivity in promoting and maintaining healthy skin for all individuals.

THE NEEDLE OF PROGRESS IS MOVING

Advances in Skin Health Equity have been increasingly significant, aiming to bridge the gaps in access to skincare resources, treatments, and education among communities worldwide. Let's take a closer look at some of the progress made within the wider industry.

The skincare industry has made strides in creating products tailored to diverse skin tones. Brands are focusing on inclusive formulations, offering a wider range of shades and addressing specific skin concerns for Melanin-Rich skin. This inclusivity in product development ensures that individuals of varying ethnicities have access to skincare that meets their specific needs.

Healthcare professionals are undergoing training to enhance cultural competency. This involves understanding the unique needs of diverse skin types, recognizing cultural influences on skincare practices, and offering personalized and respectful care to individuals from different ethnic backgrounds.

Initiatives promoting skin health education and awareness among marginalized communities have expanded. Outreach programs, campaigns, and online resources provide accessible information about skincare, sun protection, and the importance of early detection of skin conditions. These efforts aim to empower individuals to take charge of their skin health and seek appropriate care. Hallelujah to that!

In 2022, 2023 and 2024 I have had the pleasure of teaming up with innovators of formulas, professional brands and skin technology leaders like SPOTMYUV, Dermalogica PRO, AlumierMD, KOA, Training Institutes in the Caribbean and North America, scores of Medi-clinics and Skin Professionals on a global scale. So I know firsthand that the needle *is* moving.

There's a growing emphasis on dermatological research that focuses on diverse skin types. Studies exploring skin conditions, treatments, and reactions to different skincare ingredients across ethnicities contribute to a more comprehensive understanding of skin health. Furthermore, efforts to increase the representation of diverse populations in clinical trials help ensure that skincare solutions are effective for everyone.

Advocacy groups and policymakers are pushing for changes that promote Skin Health Equity. This includes advocating for more affordable and accessible skincare options, addressing disparities in dermatological care, and pushing for policies that encourage diversity and inclusivity within the skincare and healthcare industries.

Grassroots initiatives are empowering communities to prioritize skin health. These initiatives involve community engagement, workshops, and support groups that encourage open discussions about skincare, dispel myths, and encourage regular check-ups, fostering a proactive approach to skin health.

Skin Professionals and Dermatologists are recognizing the importance of diversity and inclusivity within their fields. Training programs focusing on diverse skin types and cultural nuances are equipping Skin Professionals with the knowledge and skills needed to provide comprehensive care to individuals from different backgrounds.

These collective efforts signify a shift towards a more inclusive, informed, and equitable approach to skin health. By addressing challenges in access, education, and representation, advancements in Skin Health Equity aim to ensure that everyone, regardless of their background, has access to effective skincare and dermatological care.

SKIN THEOLOGIAN'S SKINSIGHT

Here's some skin health equity progress that I've loved:

• Unilever R&D's Polycultural Centre of Excellence developing products to address the unmet needs in the beauty, wellbeing and personal care space. Combining an industry-leading understanding of Melanin-Rich skin with insights from Dermatologists and consumers of color.

• Vogue Business naming Melanin-Rich skin care as beauty's next big opportunity.

• The American Academy of Dermatology launched their Skin of Color Curriculum training.

• "Melanin-safe" skincare seeing growing recognition within the industry

• Google launched a more inclusive alternative to the Fitzpatrick Scale, revealing the Monk Skin Tone Scale.

• Work by the University of Manchester and major retailers on Skin Health Equity.

In more specific terms here are some of the tremendous collaborations I partnered with:

• Dermalogica PRO's tremendous work around Melanin-Rich skin. Their FREE and ever-green online training for Skin Professionals at www.treatingmelaninrichskin.com

Also, I've worked with their markets in Australia, Belgium, The Netherlands, The U.S., Canada and South Africa.

• At IMCAS-Paris World Congress 2024, I partnered with Dermalogica PRO's Innovation team, industry-leading Dermatologists and experts to speak on the medical-aesthetic approaches & uniquenesses of Melanin-Rich skin.

• SPOTMYUV on their innovation of a product to detect re-application time for UV protection for all skin tones, with great emphasis on Melanin-Rich skin.

• The KAO Corporation and Salon Team for their exceptional efforts in diversity and inclusivity at the consultation experience level of clients with Melanin-Rich skin and Textured Hair.

All are committed to "Sustainable Equity".

THERE'S STILL WORK TO BE DONE

Setbacks, missed opportunities, and the continual presence of inauthentic change in Skin Health Equity represent ongoing challenges and shortcomings in achieving fairness and inclusivity in skincare and dermatological care.

It still pains me to talk about this, but it's part of the process of growth, progress and development. Here's some of the not-so-great news when it comes to equity in the skin space.

Despite efforts to promote Skin Health Equity, disparities persist. Access to adequate skincare resources, dermatological care, and information remains unequal among various groups and marginalized communities. Economic barriers, geographical disparities, and lack of Cultural Intelligence all contribute to these ongoing discrepancies.

There's a continuing lack of representation and inclusivity in skincare research, clinical trials, and product development. This absence leads to a lack of understanding of diverse skin types and the specific needs of different ethnicities, resulting in limited access to effective treatments and skin care tailored to various skin tones.

Clients with Melanin-Rich skin are *still* being turned away from Skin treatment centers due to systemic business model inequities.

In some instances, efforts towards Skin Health Equity might be perceived as superficial or tokenistic. Cosmetic diversity or inclusivity campaigns without real, authentic changes in product offerings or healthcare practices can lead to inauthentic changes that fail to address underlying disparities or improve access to equitable skincare solutions.

Educational outreach and accessible information on skincare practices and conditions for some populations remain inadequate. This leads to a lack of awareness about specific skincare needs, preventive measures, and available treatments within various communities, hindering proactive skin health practices.

A lack of Cultural Intelligence among Skin Pros and healthcare providers contributes to the continuation of inequities. Yes, there have been huge swings in the right direction but unfortunately, we aren't quite there yet. Insufficient understanding of cultural nuances in skincare practices and inadequate communication with diverse populations may result in less-than-ideal care and missed opportunities for tailored treatment plans.

Economic disparities and accessibility issues in accessing quality skincare products, treatments, and dermatological consultations - that are suitable for clients with Melanin-Rich skin - still persist. Limited availability of affordable and accessible skincare resources can create barriers for individuals from marginalized communities to accessing essential skincare.

Addressing these setbacks and creating authentic change in Skin Health Equity requires concerted efforts. Meaning it literally takes a village. No one individual, company, chemist or professional can do it all. It involves promoting genuine inclusivity in research, curriculum, product development, and healthcare practices, advocating for policies that support equitable access, enhancing Cultural Intelligence practices, and ensuring representation and diversity in all facets of skin care and dermatological care.

DIVERSITY & INCLUSIVITY BEAUTY EXPERT INSIGHTS

I asked Diversity in Beauty Expert Maria Michelle Lee for her insights on diversity and inclusivity in the industry.

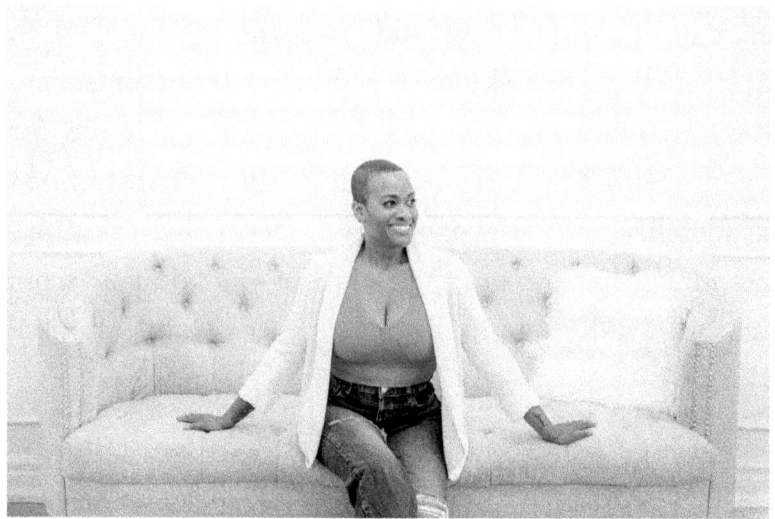

Here's what she had to say:

"We have come a long way over the past 30 years. In the sunless tanning industry, I work in, it was unheard of that people with Melanin-Rich skin would choose spray tans.

There was also a lack of education on sun damage and how to prevent it, as well as the sunless options available. Now with the help of social media, better education and more support from brands like Sephora, it's becoming more normalized. Anyone who wants a spray tan, for whatever reason, can feel confident and comfortable getting one.

As a Diversity In Beauty Expert, a big challenge was not only being seen but being heard. We are not a trend, we are a diverse group of people who have Melanin-Rich skin tones and diverse backgrounds.

It's still about education. The challenge is making sure that there is a known difference in the depth, tone, and texture of our skin and that all aesthetic equipment and products shouldn't be marketed/offered as inclusive to all skin types, as all skin types are not the same.

Pay is also a problem. The marketing dollars are there but they are not shared equally in my opinion. There are still professionals who have Melanin-Rich skin who aren't being paid appropriately. This needs to change.

WHY SUSTAINABLE EQUITY IS SO IMPORTANT

Rather than focusing on short-term strategies, tokenism and half-measures, I think the key to true change and Skin Health Equity is actually sustaining it.

What do I mean by that? Well, here goes. Sustainable equity in skincare is about efforts to make the industry more inclusive and culturally aware in a sustainable way. That means implementing long-term strategies, policies and practices that ensure equitable access to skincare resources, treatments and representation for individuals from all backgrounds.

This goes way beyond short-term initiatives and cosmetic changes, emphasizing the need for continuous commitment to genuine inclusivity and industry-wide changes.

Sustainable equity in skincare involves creating an environment where diversity is valued, diverse voices are heard and meaningful actions are taken to address inequality in access and representation within the skincare space.

WHAT'S THE PROBLEM?

Short-lived efforts, such as the establishment of diversity and inclusion (D&I) departments within the industry can sometimes lack meaningful impact - which means nothing *really* changes, even though it looks like a step in the right direction.

It could be that those appointed to tackle these issues may lack adequate support, diverse representation within the company's leadership or the budget to drive substantial change.

But really? It's about money. There, I said it.

To achieve sustainable equity, skincare companies need to move beyond performative actions and commit to genuine structural changes. This involves creating a thriving culture of inclusivity from top to bottom along with supportive policies, and practices.

It requires diverse representation at all levels of the organization, ensuring that voices from all backgrounds contribute to decision-making processes, from product development to marketing strategies. In the US less than 3% of Dermatologists are Black, with a population where 40% are Melanin-Rich.[2]

It also means investing in training programs that enhance cultural competency among Skin Professionals. This equips them with the skills and understanding needed to provide effective and inclusive care to individuals from all cultural backgrounds. This improves the industry for the people working in and using it.

Continual evaluation and assessment of progress are also essential to create sustainable equity in skincare. It's too easy to set it and forget it when it comes to implementing these changes - unless it's that rare occasion when it makes it to the external stage for some good publicity (I promise I'm not a cynic but I've seen this happen far too often for my liking).

My professional opinion is this: Companies should establish benchmarks to measure the impact of their initiatives, making sure that these efforts result in real improvements in access, representation and inclusivity.

This ongoing monitoring helps to identify the areas that aren't quite there yet.

Ultimately, sustainable equity in skincare demands an all-around, enduring commitment to diversity, inclusivity and equitable practices. It's about creating an environment where inclusivity is not just a trend or a short-term initiative but an integral part of the company's values, operations, and dedication to providing accessible and effective skincare for everyone, regardless of their background.

SKIN THEOLOGIAN'S SKINSIGHT

In 2022, Neutrogena announced its "Heroes of Skin Health Equity" initiative, the brand's latest effort aimed at improving skin health equity for those with Black and brown skin.

This was exciting as it championed those looking to make a difference when it came to skin health equity.

However, it doesn't look as though the initiative made it to 2023 or 2024, which is a little disappointing. This shows just how important it is that Skin Health Equity is done intentionally.

IT'S TIME TO LEVEL-UP TRAINING

The industry has often faced criticism for inadequate training in promoting Skin Health Equity. I'm talking from the undergraduate level with Academies, Institutes and other formal places of learning. Many qualifying Skin Professionals receive insufficient education on diverse skin types, cultural nuances, and the specific needs of clients, leading to gaps in understanding and care.

There's often a lack of how to work with all skin types, tones and shades. This leads to Skin Pros who are out in the industry feeling uncomfortable working on Melanin-Rich skin. It is this lack of confidence that feeds the cycle of clients who have Melanin-Rich skin having a poor experience, misconceptions and limited treatment options.

This is also how we end up with stereotypes and biases in skin care practices, further blocking true Skin Health Equity within the industry.

There's a pressing need for enhanced educational curriculums and ongoing training opportunities that prioritize cultural competency, diversity, and inclusivity within the beauty industry. This ensures that Skin Pros are equipped with the knowledge and skills necessary to provide effective, respectful, and tailored care to clients of all ethnicities and backgrounds.

SOME TECH HAS IMPROVED BUT CHALLENGES STILL REMAIN

Beauty tech's failure to cater to Melanin-Rich skin stems from a few different things.

The main reason is a lack of representation in the development and testing phases of beauty technology. Most beauty tech innovations are conceived and tested on limited skin types, often favoring lighter complexions, which leads to products and tools that might not effectively address the unique concerns of Melanin-Rich skin. Some might even cause damage to Melanin-Rich skin.

Another critical aspect is the absence of diverse datasets in training algorithms for skincare and beauty tech. Artificial intelligence and machine learning, pivotal in many beauty tech applications, heavily rely on databases for training.

Unfortunately, these datasets often lack diversity, resulting in algorithms that struggle to recognize, analyze or provide accurate recommendations for darker skin tones.

Preconceived notions and biases against darker skin tones may influence product development, where innovations might overlook or misinterpret the distinct characteristics and needs of individuals with Melanin-Rich skin.

It's also about money. Let's face it, the beauty tech industry might prioritize markets that they perceive as larger or more profitable, often overlooking the needs of smaller, underserved demographics, including Melanin-Rich communities.

Moreover, the lack of diversity within the teams developing beauty tech solutions is a significant barrier. Without diverse representation in product design and decision-making roles, the nuanced needs of diverse skin tones may not be adequately considered during the development and testing phases.

There's an opportunity here - to design and create this technology with teams who have lived experience of being Melanin-Rich and in the beauty space. The algorithms need to be built with a diverse range of experience, recognition and acknowledgement in there so that we end up with a beauty space that's suitable for everyone.

3

MELANIN-RICH AI: HOW AND WHY?

By leveraging advanced algorithms, AI systems can identify and mitigate biases...

I n this chapter, you'll see:

- How AI is being used in the skincare industry
- What this use of AI means for those with Melanin-Rich skin
- CQ opportunities that AI could influence

ME, MYSELF AND AI

Let's start with what AI actually is. AI, or Artificial Intelligence, refers to the simulation of human intelligence in machines that are programmed to think, learn, and problem-solve like humans. The goal of AI is to develop systems that can perform tasks that typically require human intelligence, such as visual perception, speech recognition, decision-making, language translation, and problem-solving.

AI is being increasingly integrated into various aspects of the skincare industry, offering innovative solutions and enhancing the overall consumer experience. Here are several ways in which AI is being utilized in the skincare sector:

AI algorithms analyze individual skin characteristics, including type, tone, and specific concerns, to provide personalized skincare recommendations. This ensures that consumers receive tailored advice and product suggestions based on their unique needs.

Virtual try-on and augmented reality (AR) applications use AI to simulate the effects of skincare products on a user's face. This allows consumers to virtually test different products before making a purchase, enhancing the online shopping experience.

Skin analysis applications use AI to evaluate images of the skin to assess conditions such as wrinkles, pigmentation, and hydration levels. Users can receive insights into their skin health and track changes over time, facilitating a more informed approach to skincare.

AI assists in analyzing vast databases of skincare ingredients and formulations, helping companies develop products that are effective and tailored to specific skin needs. This accelerates the formulation process and promotes the creation of innovative and science-backed skincare solutions. There are some cosmetic chemists who query the accuracy of AI when it comes to developing and formulating new products.

Chatbots and virtual assistants are using AI to provide instant customer support, answer skincare-related queries, and offer guidance on product usage. This enhances customer engagement and satisfaction while addressing concerns in real time.

AI is also being used in the business and logistics side of skincare - such as supporting marketing activities, optimizing the supply chain, predicting trends and helping with clinical diagnosis and treatment planning.

As technology continues to advance, AI is likely to play an increasingly integral role in shaping the future of skincare, offering innovative solutions, improving product effectiveness, and enhancing the overall consumer experience.

AI'S PRECISION IN UNDERSTANDING MELANIN-RICH SKIN

One of the challenges with AI is that it's only as good as the inputs it has. Often those inputs come from the information that the algorithms find in 'real life'. And as we've already identified (multiple times, across multiple books - you know the drill by now), most resources aren't quite up to speed.

This means that the biases, misinformation and lack of information are taken from existing educational resources and carried through to AI-generated educational resources, skin analysis tools and information. And so the cycle continues (sigh).

AI provides analysis of melanin levels and other skin characteristics through advanced algorithms. These algorithms process vast amounts of data, enabling accurate assessments of melanin distribution, pigmentation, and other key features, contributing to a more nuanced understanding of diverse skin types.

The potential for AI to revolutionize the initial assessment stage in skincare practices is immense. By streamlining and enhancing the accuracy of skin analysis, AI ensures that Skin Professionals have a comprehensive understanding of individual needs from the outset. This not only improves the efficiency of skincare practices but also sets the stage for personalized and effective treatment plans.

However, remember, the algorithms are only as good as the data that is being input into them. If these AI models are being trained on one type of skin only, or a proportion of society that isn't representative, then there won't be a representative sample for AI algorithms to learn from.

AI'S ROLE IN MITIGATING BIAS AND FOSTERING INCLUSIVITY

The skincare industry has historically grappled with biases embedded in traditional algorithms, which often fail to account for the diversity of skin types. These biases can manifest in various forms, from inaccuracies in diagnostics to the limited effectiveness of skincare products across different skin tones. The prevalence of such biases highlights a critical need for a more inclusive and accurate approach to skincare, prompting the exploration of AI as a transformative solution.

By leveraging advanced algorithms, AI systems can identify and mitigate biases, leading to more precise and equitable assessments of skin conditions. These studies demonstrate the potential for AI to serve as a corrective force, steering the skincare industry toward fairness and accuracy in its treatment recommendations.

AI algorithms not only have the capability to rectify biases but also contribute to fair representation of diverse skin tones. Stories abound of AI systems successfully adapting and providing accurate analyses for individuals with melanin-rich skin, previously underrepresented or misjudged by traditional algorithms. This shift toward inclusivity reinforces the idea that AI has the potential to revolutionize skincare by embracing the diversity inherent in global populations.

An essential component of combating biases in skincare algorithms lies in the cultivation of unbiased training datasets for AI. Narratives emphasize the significance of incorporating diverse and representative data during the training process to ensure that AI algorithms learn from a broad spectrum of skin types. In this way, the skincare industry can foster more equitable AI applications, ultimately contributing to a more inclusive and effective approach to skincare for individuals of all backgrounds.

AI systems can exhibit bias, including racial bias, depending on how they are trained and the data they are exposed to during their development. If the training data used to teach an AI model is not diverse or representative, the model may not perform well across various demographics, including different skin tones.

Historically, there have been instances where AI systems, such as facial recognition algorithms, showed bias against people with darker skin tones. This bias is often attributed to imbalances in the training data, with lighter skin tones being overrepresented. In such cases, the AI system may struggle to accurately recognize or analyze features in individuals with darker skin.

Efforts are being made to address these biases and improve the fairness and inclusivity of AI systems. It is crucial for developers to use diverse datasets that represent the full spectrum of human characteristics. Additionally, ongoing research and scrutiny are essential to identify and rectify biases in AI algorithms to ensure fair and unbiased performance across all demographic groups.

If you encounter instances of bias, it's important to raise awareness and advocate for improvements in AI technologies to mitigate these issues.

SKIN THEOLOGIAN'S SKINSIGHT

If you're more familiar with AI than the average person, then chances are you've heard of ChatGPT. It's a chatbot developed by OpenAI and launched on November 30, 2022. Based on a large language model, it enables users to refine and steer a conversation towards a desired length, format, style, level of detail and language.

Basically, it's somewhere between a search engine, information tool and chatbot. It delivers information it finds online in a more user-friendly and relatable way.

A Skin Pro might use a tool like ChatGPT to help them create educational, social or website content. They may use it to support their client consultations, admin services or research. Two things to remember are that AI tools don't always have access to the latest information, and sometimes when it doesn't know the answer to what it's being asked, it fills in the gaps with its best guess. And that's not always accurate.

Like most AI-driven tools, it learns from what's already out there online. And some of that demonstrates racial bias, stereotypes and overt racism. Dare I say, even at times, a subjective approach and view, rather than an objective, curated one. ChatGPT's creators have built in some systems to stop overtly racist content from being creative, but unfortunately, there are workarounds if you're determined to make it take on a biased approach to the content it creates.

Let me introduce you to Erin Reddick - the Founder of ChatBlackGPT™ and Certified Prompt Engineer, AI Developer and Entrepreneur.

Yes, I'm standing up and clapping on this one, because when I learnt of her expertise and AI launch, I was immensely elated and knew I needed to share this.

Allow me to add... No, this is not a collaboration, as I don't know Miss Reddick nor will I receive any percentage on any service, products, brands or companies mentioned in this or any of my works. It's simply because these needed to be talked about. No gate-keeping here.

She developed an AI tool that speaks from a culturally aware perspective of those with

Melanin-Rich skin. That tool is ChatBlackGPT™.

It's been designed to produce data, insights and perspectives from Black, African American and African information sources only. It answers from a Black perspective, adopting a response style that reflects cultural awareness, sensitivity, and respect.

The difference between the way this tool responds vs the original ChatGPT is noticeable, refreshing and a huge stride forward when it comes to progressing AI tools to be inclusive.

Yes, this can bring to question, "What about other cultures and backgrounds?" To that I say, I can't speak, but I do know this is a phenomenal step in the right direction for great disparities in representation historically. I hope you give it a go in your continual professional and personal growth.

AI AND SKIN EDUCATION

AI can be harnessed to enhance education in skincare, particularly in areas related to cultural intelligence and diversity. Let's take a closer look at how it can be utilized to support much-needed goals in skincare education.

Virtual simulations and AR applications powered by AI can provide students with hands-on, immersive experiences. This allows them to practice skincare techniques on virtual models with diverse skin tones, helping to develop practical skills while promoting cultural intelligence and sensitivity.

AI can be used to develop training modules that focus on cultural sensitivity in skin care practices. These modules can include information on diverse beauty standards, traditional skincare rituals, and cultural considerations when interacting with clients from different backgrounds.

AI algorithms can also be used to analyze and curate case studies that represent a diverse range of skin types and cultural backgrounds. This helps students understand the variations in skincare needs and practices across different ethnicities, promoting a more comprehensive and inclusive education.

OPPORTUNITIES FOR AI TO SUPPORT CQ

AI technology has the potential to contribute significantly to making skincare more inclusive. Here's how:

For example, it can analyze vast datasets that include a wide range of skin types and tones. By doing so, AI-powered skincare platforms can provide more accurate and personalized recommendations that cater to the unique needs of individuals with different skin characteristics. This ensures that skincare products and routines are more inclusive and effective for diverse populations.

While AI holds great promise for making skincare more inclusive, it's crucial to ensure that the technology is developed and implemented with careful consideration of ethical and fairness principles. Efforts to diversify datasets, address biases, and prioritize inclusivity in AI applications can collectively contribute to a more equitable and accessible skincare landscape.

EMERGING TECH AND FUTURE TRENDS

The skincare industry is changing with new technologies. More people are using AI for virtual dermatology consultations, making it easier for them to get personalized skincare advice. The numbers show a big increase in the use of these virtual consultations, making skincare guidance accessible to a broader audience.

In the future, we can expect more collaboration between AI and skincare professionals. This teamwork leads to ongoing improvements in how skin care is done. Stories of successful collaborations show that AI can provide valuable insights, helping professionals create better and more personalized treatment plans.

Studies on innovative AI technologies are also showing how the future of skincare is changing, especially for Melanin-Rich skin care. AI is being used to address specific concerns related to different skin types, making skincare more inclusive and effective. Overall, AI is making skincare more accessible, personalized, and effective, transforming the industry for the better.

4

MELANOCYTES: THE GOOD | THE BAD | THE SCIENCE

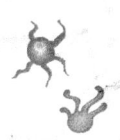

Let's go back to the absolute beginning.

I n this chapter, you'll explore:

- Melanocytes and why they're important for Melanin-Rich skin
- How melanocytes work
- What happens when melanocytes are neglected or damaged

WHAT IS MELANIN?

Now it's time for us to get into the heart of Melanin: where it lives. I know. You're excited for this one.

Melanin is a pigment produced by specialized cells called melanocytes found in the skin, hair follicles, and eyes. It's the substance responsible for the color of our skin, hair, and irises. This pigment is what gives our skin its diverse range of tones.

Melanin is extremely important as a protective function in the body. When our skin is exposed to sunlight, melanocytes kick into action, producing more melanin as a natural defense mechanism against harmful UV rays.

It acts as a shield, absorbing and scattering the UV radiation before it can penetrate deep into the skin and cause damage. This protection helps prevent sunburns, skin aging, and the development of skin cancers like melanoma.

But before you get too excited, this isn't cellular immutability.

New research[1] confirms that the level of protection that Melanocytes produce when foreign UV rays enter is irrelevant to the degree of damage being incurred in the skin. Your skin will still end up being damaged and prone to serious skin concerns.

There are two primary types of melanin — Eumelanin and Pheomelanin. Eumelanin comes in brown and black hues and provides more photoprotection, while Pheomelanin is responsible for red and yellow pigments and offers less protection against UV rays. [See Fig. 1.]

Eumelanin is less soluble than Pheomelanin, which can make it more difficult to treat. Both types of melanin can be treated, but skin which has more Eumelanin takes more time to treat when it comes to skin concerns. Since hyperpigmentation is the primary concern in clients with Melanin-Rich skin, Skin Pros must be equipped with the appropriate tools, technology and formulations to address it effectively.

The production and distribution of these melanin-influencing types determine our skin's color and its response to sunlight, showcasing the vital role melanin plays in both our appearance and our skin's defense mechanisms against sun damage.

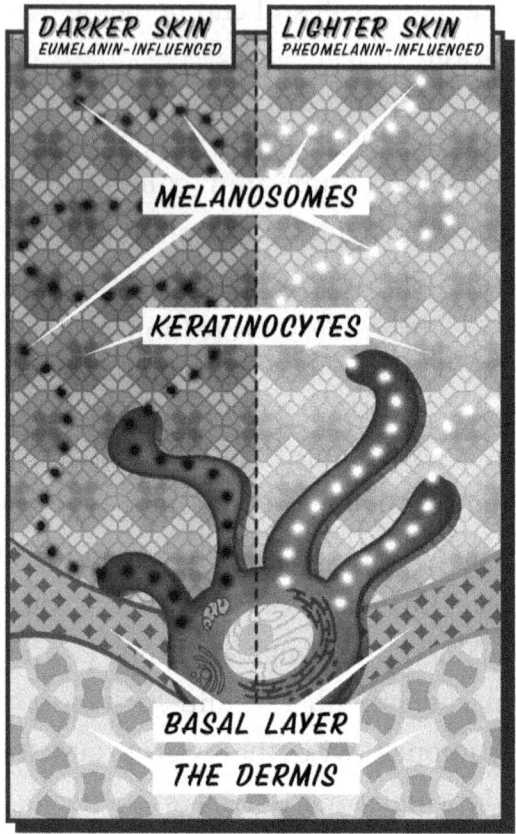

[Fig. 1.]

UNRIDDLING THE MELANOCYTE

Let's go back to the absolute beginning of Melanin-Rich skin.

The melanocyte.

It's basically one of the building blocks of your skin.

Melanocytes are specialized cells found in your skin, hair, and eyes that are responsible for producing the pigment in your skin (aka melanin). Within the skin, melanocytes live in the bottom layer of the Epidermis, called the Stratum Germinativum, or the Stratum Basale (Basal Layer).

These cells hang out in the deeper layers of your skin and work like tiny color factories, creating melanin that gives your skin its natural tone, helping protect it from the sun's harmful rays, and determining your hair and eye color too. Essentially, they're the masterminds behind your unique appearance.

Understanding their structure, functions, and immune roles is key to appreciating their significance in maintaining skin health - especially when it comes to Melanin-Rich skin.

THE BUILDING BLOCKS OF MELANOCYTES

Melanocytes aren't alone; they cozy up in the epidermal layer, typically at the basal layer—the deepest layer of the epidermis. They're quite distinctive, with long, branch-like projections that extend among neighboring skin cells. These branch-like projections are called Dendrites, which is significant to how various formula ingredients work to influence this cell. More on that soon.

These cells don't just sit around. They're basically where melanin production occurs. Picture tiny containers within the cell, housing the melanin pigment in varying amounts, dictating the skin's coloration.

The tiny containers that the melanin is housed in are called Melanosomes. They travel up through the Dendrites, delivering pigment to approximately 36 other surrounding cells. These surrounding cells are called Corneocytes or Keratinocytes. On average there are 10 Corneocytes to 1 Melanocyte. So clearly, we see that the Melanocytes go to work!

How Dendrites transfer the melanosomes to the neighboring cells is still inconclusive. Chemists theorize that it is via Phagocytosis. Others say, a level of Mitosis, while others lean towards literal depositing. However melanin is transferred, we know it is just that; transferred!

[See Fig. 2.]

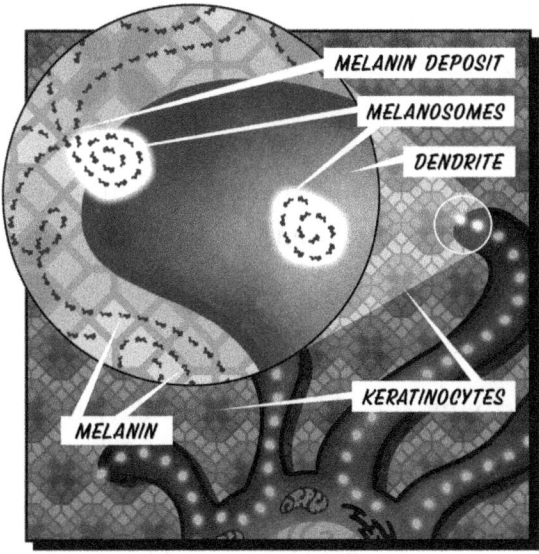

[Fig. 2.]

Almost everyone - with the exception of some conditions such as albinism - has melanin in their skin, whatever their shade or tone. It's just that the influence of Eumelanin or Pheomelanin in the skin determines the quality of melanin and what that tone is.

These specialist cells synthesize melanin through a complex process involving enzymes like L-DOPA, Tyrosinase and Tyrosine. L-DOPA acts like a building block for making melanin, through a process guided by an enzyme called Tyrosinase. Tyrosinase is an essential enzyme for melanin synthesis within melanocytes whereas Tyrosine is an amino acid that's used in the process of producing melanin. The body also uses the mineral Copper as part of the process. This complex yet brilliant process is referred to as the Tyrosinase cascade.

The end-point of pigment production is a form of protection. When exposed to sunlight, melanocytes kick into gear, producing more melanin to shield the skin from harmful UV rays.

This is also why the skin becomes darker or changes after UV exposure (stimulant). It's also why some skin concerns like melasma and hyperpigmentation show up after spending time in the sun. A tan is actually your skin trying to save itself from damage.

Incidentally, a version of this mechanism happens in the affected region whenever the melanocyte cell is stimulated by other triggers that inflame the skin. Think bug bites, deep acne breakouts and hormonal skin changes.

But back to UV exposure. Melanocytes aren't just about skin tones. As mentioned above, they distribute melanin to neighboring skin cells, the keratinocytes, offering them UV protection as well. This teamwork is what gives our skin its color and works to defend the nucleus from detrimental damage.

Just FYI keratinocytes are the main cells that make up the epidermis, the outermost layer of the skin. These specialized cells make up about 90% of the epidermis and play a crucial role in maintaining the skin's integrity and barrier function.

Their primary function is to produce keratin, a tough, fibrous protein that forms the structural framework of the skin, hair, and nails. As keratinocytes move upwards through the layers of the epidermis, they undergo a process called differentiation, transforming into flattened, hardened cells filled with keratin.

These cells eventually form the protective outer layer of the skin, providing strength, resilience, and protection against environmental factors like UV radiation, microbes, and physical damage. Keratinocytes also contribute to wound healing by rapidly dividing to replace damaged or lost skin cells, ensuring the skin's continuous renewal and repair.

Just a little context there for how melanocytes and keratinocytes work together in the skin. Anyway, back to focusing on those all-important melanocytes.

Think melanocytes are done and dusted there? Nope. Melanocytes moonlight as immune defenders too. They play a role in the skin's immune responses, communicating with other immune cells when necessary. This helps in managing inflammatory responses and defending against potential threats.

Did you know that dendritic cells within the Epidermis, due to their complexity, hold the potential for mutations that lead to cancer? The dendritic family includes the Langerhans cell (living in the Squamous layer), the Merkel cell and the Melanocyte cell (both living in the Basal layer). All of these cells, due to their dendritic sensitivities to foreign substances are potential starting points for skin cancers. I.e. Squamous Cell Carcinoma (SCC), Basal Cell Carcinoma (BCC) & Merkel Cell Carcinoma (MCC).

SKIN THEOLOGIAN'S SKINSIGHT

You might be wondering why you need to care about inflammation, especially when it comes to deeper skin tones.

Uncontrolled inflammation is bad news for all skin tones, especially Melanin-Rich skin. It poses unique challenges for darker skin due to its potential to trigger post-inflammatory hyperpigmentation (PIH).

When darker skin tones undergo uncontrolled inflammation—due to factors like acne, injury, or irritation—there's an increased risk of developing PIH. PIH manifests as darkened patches or spots in areas previously affected by trauma or injury.

A study in the Journal of Drugs and Dermatology[2] found that acne, dry skin and dark spots (aka hyperpigmentation) were the top concerns for people with Melanin-Rich skin. So it makes sense to understand it, so it can be avoided.

The melanocytes, responsible for producing melanin, respond more robustly to inflammatory signals in dark skin. This heightened response can lead to excessive melanin production and uneven distribution, resulting in discoloration after the initial inflammation has healed.

Compared to lighter skin tones, this hyperpigmentation is more visible and can take longer to fade in dark skin. Friendly reminder of the insolubility of Eumelanin that we mentioned earlier.

See below [Fig. 3.] and [Fig.4.]

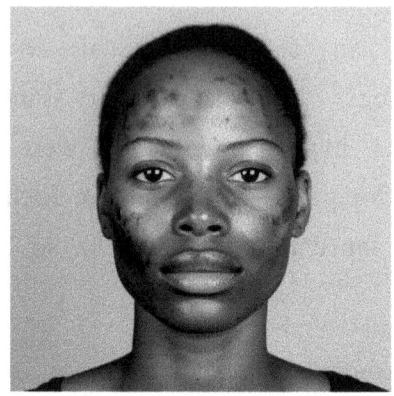

[Fig. 3]

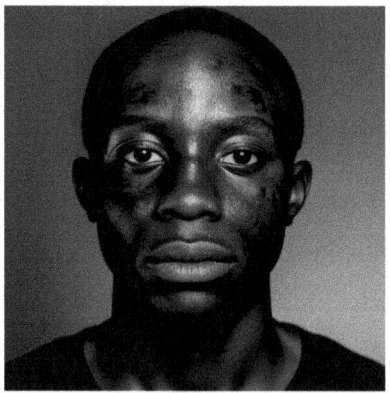

[Fig. 4]

While inflammation is a natural response to injury or irritation in all skin tones, it's particularly concerning for Melanin-Rich skin due to the increased probability of PIH.

Managing inflammation promptly and employing skincare strategies to minimize its impact can help reduce the risk of PIH in individuals with Melanin-Rich skin.

Inflammation is also uncomfortable and can be noticeable so it's definitely something that you want to avoid for clients wherever possible.

Research[3] has shown that hyperpigmentation, acne and inflammation are all connected from the earliest stages of acne development. It can be considered as 'persistent' rather than 'post-inflammatory' in some cases because the underlying inflammation may still be present even if it doesn't seem to be visible on the surface.

They also produce antimicrobial peptides,[4] adding another layer of defense against microbial invaders. The study submits that skin with darker-quality melanin is less susceptible to some microorganisms and bacteria than lighter-quality melanin. It's fascinating just how much of an impact melanocytes can have on your skin overall.

UNDERSTANDING CONSTITUTIVE AND FACULTATIVE COLOR

Keep your seat because I'm about to hit you with some more skin science. I'll start out with a quick explanation and then we'll move into how this fits in with melanocytes.

The title of this section refers to why our skin tone is what it is and why our skin tone can change a little. Constitutive and facultative skin colors essentially mean the different ways our skin gets its pigmentation.

Constitutive color is your natural, inherent skin tone—the color you're born with and is determined by your genetics. It's the baseline shade that you carry without any external influences.

Facultative color, on the other hand, is influenced by external factors like sun exposure, hormonal changes, other environmental elements or trauma, leading to PIH. [Figures 3 & 4.].

When you spend time in the sun and your skin gets darker - that's facultative color in action. It's a temporary change in pigmentation due to external factors and doesn't alter your natural constitutive color permanently.

The significance of melanocyte cells goes beyond just looks and skin tones too. Neglecting melanocyte health can have serious consequences.

Damaged or dysfunctional melanocytes, such as pendulous melanocytes can lead to skin conditions like vitiligo (loss of skin pigmentation) or, worse, contribute to the development of skin cancers, including melanoma - the most dangerous form of skin cancer.

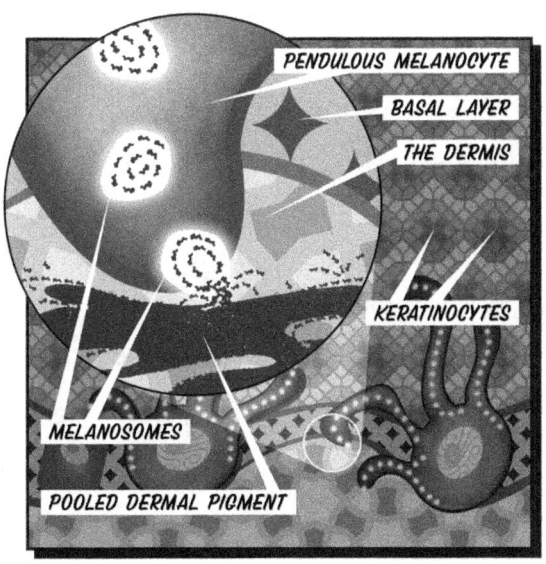

[Fig. 5]

This can also lead to dermal hyper-pigmentation which is not treatable with conventional approaches. Since the epidermis is constantly renewing, hyper-pigmentation in the epidermis eventually migrates upwards and off of the skin. However, if the Dendrite has a pendulum swing downwards (i.e. pendulous) -[See Fig. 5.], the pigment is pooled into the Dermis. So hyper-pigmentation stays in the Papillary layer of the Dermis as 'pooled melanin' and does not fade. Determining whether pigmentation is dermal or epidermal is significant for Skin Pros.

Try these 3 tips to be able to determine whether hyper-pigmentation is epidermal or dermal.

- **Tip #1:** Ask how long the hyper-pigmentation has been there.
- **Tip #2:** Utilize a Skin Scanner or black light technology to peer beyond the naked eye's ability to see hyper-pigmentation.
- **Tip #3:** Determine if the area has been treated before with minimal improvement.

SKIN THEOLOGIAN'S SKINSIGHT

Encouraging constitutive color, or the natural color of our skin determined by genetics, is important for a few reasons.

Firstly, it celebrates and respects the inherent beauty of diverse skin tones. Embracing and preserving our natural color promotes inclusivity and appreciation for the spectrum of skin shades within our society (which - no surprise - is hugely important to me).

When I talk about encouraging our natural color, I mean we want to keep the skin healthy and happy without disturbance to the melanocytes.

These cells are superheroes—they protect the skin from UV light. But sometimes they can go a bit overboard, making too much pigment and causing skin issues. So, we want to make sure they're doing their job right.

By preserving natural color and being careful in the sun, like using sunscreen and wearing protective clothes, we keep our skin healthy and reduce the chances of problems like skin damage or even skin cancer.

And it goes without saying - but I'm gonna say it just in case you forgot - keep an eye on your skin, and the skin of your clients if you're a Skin Pro.

Check it and take notice of anything that's unusual, new or just doesn't feel right. Don't be afraid to go to the doctor (sooner rather than later) and take measurements or photos if you're concerned.

It could quite literally save your skin, and your life.

Melanoma and Skin Health Threats

Melanoma is a type of skin cancer that originates in the melanocytes. It's often considered the most dangerous form of skin cancer because it can spread to other parts of the body quickly if not detected and treated early.

Melanin-Rich skin is far *less* likely to develop melanoma than non-Hispanic White skin (at a rate of 1 per 100,000 compared to 30 per 100,000) due to the protection that melanin provides from damaging ultraviolet rays.

However, individuals who have Melanin-Rich skin who do develop this type of cancer have a much lower five-year survival rate. From 2011 through 2015, the five-year survival rate in the United States for Black patients was 66% compared with 90% for non-Hispanic White patients, according to a 2019 study published by the Centers for Disease Control and Prevention.[5]

The reality is that there are lots of misconceptions about Melanin-Rich skin, even within the Melanin-Rich communities. Darker skin tones can - unfortunately - experience skin cancers, including melanoma. We'll highlight a specific type below.

Melanoma originates from melanocytes in your skin cells turning rogue, dividing uncontrollably and potentially spreading to other parts of the body. This makes early detection crucial, as advanced melanoma can be life-threatening.

Acral Lentiginous Melanoma (ALM)

Acral lentiginous melanoma (ALM) is a form of melanoma. The word "acral" is Greek meaning "extremity" referring to the furthest parts from the center of the body (hands and feet). "Lentiginous" refers to the darkened pigment that shows up. This type of melanoma typically appears on the palms of the hands, soles of the feet, or underneath the nails. It accounts for around 5-10% of all melanoma cases - so it's rare but tends to be pretty aggressive.

Although it's less common compared to other types of melanoma, it tends to disproportionately affect individuals with deeper skin tones.

Studies suggest that ALM is more prevalent among people of Asian, African, and Hispanic descent. AKA, the people who tend to have more melanin in their skin. The prognoses in these individuals are more advanced at presentation due to delays in diagnosis.

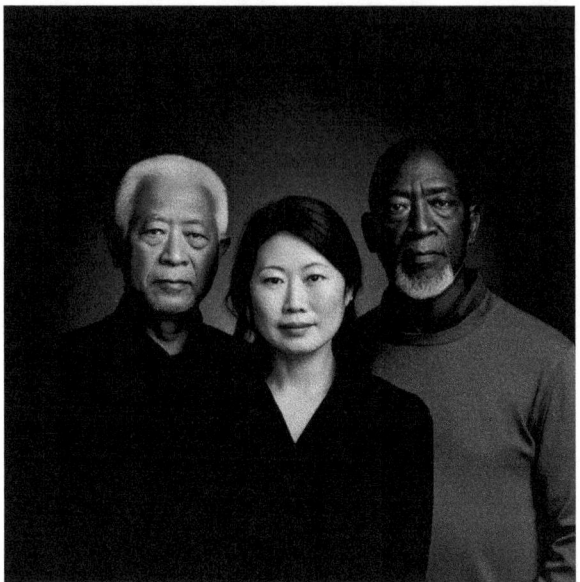

[Fig. 6.]

Unlike other forms of melanoma that may be linked to sun exposure, ALM often occurs in areas not commonly exposed to sunlight. It's more prevalent in individuals with darker skin tones, making it particularly significant to recognize and diagnose early in Melanin-Rich skin.

Identifying ALM in Melanin-Rich skin can be tricky. It might look like a dark patch or spot that seems out of place, like a stubborn bruise or a funny-colored mole on your hands or feet. Sometimes, it can be tough to spot because it doesn't follow the typical rules of pigmentary changes.

You should also be aware of the ABCDE's of abnormal skin growths. If a skin growth has any of the following, or you have any history or reason to be concerned, you need to get it checked out as soon as possible:

- A - Asymmetrical in shape
- B - Uneven Border
- C - Varying Colors
- D - Diameter is close to an eraser on a pencil
- E - Evolving or Elevating (changing)

One of the reasons why it sometimes doesn't get spotted until it's at a later stage is that it doesn't present as you might expect. Along with the myths that skin cancer doesn't affect those with Melanin-Rich skin. ALM might also present at a later stage, which can be challenging.

Keeping an eye out for any changes in texture, color, or new spots on palms, soles, or nails is important for your clients and your own health. Even small changes that seem odd or don't heal as they should are worth checking out.

If something seems off or suspicious, it's time to take a trip to your doctor or Dermatologist. Don't put it off. Even if it turns out it's nothing to worry about, it's worth getting checked just to keep your mind at ease.

And if it is something more sinister, it can be caught early, managed and treated - especially in Melanin-Rich skin where these changes might not stand out as much.

Because of its unique characteristics and challenges in identification, there's ongoing research to better understand and improve the diagnosis and treatment of ALM, especially in populations with higher Melanin-Rich skin. In medicine newer treatment modalities like immunotherapies for advanced ALM are offering promising preliminary results.

Melanin and Skin Conditions

Melanin isn't just something that can contribute to skin cancer. There are other skin conditions that are affected by melanin, melanocytes or a lack thereof, these include:

Hyperpigmentation

Excessive melanin production leads to dark patches or spots on the skin, known as hyperpigmentation. Conditions like melasma, post-inflammatory hyperpigmentation (PIH), and age spots (lentigines) often result from increased melanin in specific areas.

This can be genetic or down to external factors, such as UV exposure, medication, stress or your general health.

Hypopigmentation

Reduced or absent melanin production causing lighter patches or areas on the skin. Conditions like vitiligo and certain types of albinism are characterized by hypopigmentation due to melanin deficiency.

These conditions are both usually medical and related to genetic mutations that affect melanin production.

Again, if you're concerned about changes to your skin, or the health of your skin, speak to a medical professional and get checked over. Don't mess around when it comes to your skin and your health.

Pigmentary Disorders within Melanin-Rich Skin You May Not Know

There are some pigmentation disorders that you might be more familiar with, especially when it comes to Melanin-Rich skin. You've probably already heard of the above skin disorders.

Here are some skin conditions and disorders that can affect Melanin-Rich skin you may not be quite as familiar with. Remember, if in doubt, refer your clients to a Dermatologist or healthcare professional who can give a medical diagnosis and support towards medical treatment if required.

Epidermal Melanosis

This condition is characterized by increased melanin in the epidermis (top layer of the skin), leading to hyperpigmentation. It can appear as brown or grayish patches on the skin.

Traditional treatments may include topical depigmenting agents such as Hydroquinone, Retinoids, and Corticosteroids.

Dermal Melanosis (Pendulous Melanocytes)

Dermal Melanosis involves the accumulation of melanin in the dermis (middle layer of the skin). Pendulous melanocytes are melanin-producing cells that have migrated into the dermis.

Unconventional treatments may include laser therapy, chemical peels or cryotherapy.

Mixed Types - Both Epidermal and Dermal Melanosis.

As you know, the rule of thumb with laser options for skin that is Melanin-Rich is to use Non-Ablative lasers. These have longer wavelengths like the Nd:YAG laser at 1064 nm and have a longer coefficient. This means the laser penetrates the skin at a depth of up to 4mm, bypassing the Melanocyte cell. Removing the risk of excessive trauma.

The treatment approach may involve a combination of traditional and unconventional methods based on the predominant features of the condition.

Hyperpigmentation at the Extensor Side of Joints

Hyperpigmentation at joints may be associated with chronic inflammation in conditions like inflammatory arthritis.

Addressing the underlying inflammatory condition is crucial. Topical treatments may include Corticosteroids, while systemic medications and lifestyle changes may also be considered.

Ashy Dermatosis

Common in Melanin-Rich skin, ashy dermatosis presents as gray or ashy patches on the skin.

Management may involve emollients, topical Corticosteroids, and avoiding potential triggers. Consultation with a dermatologist is essential.

Nevus of Ota and Nevus of Ito

These are congenital, benign pigmented lesions. Nevus of Ota appears on the face, while Nevus of Ito occurs on the shoulder.

Laser therapy is often used for cosmetic purposes. However, due to the nature of these nevi, monitoring for changes is essential.

Lentigo Solaris

Also known as solar lentigines, sun spots or age spots, lentigo solaris results from sun exposure and appears as flat, brown or black spots. Yes, Melanin-Rich Skin does get sun spots, albeit, not as obvious as in lighter skin.

Beyond referring to them as sun spots, recognizing the potential for malignancy is crucial. Treatment may include cryotherapy, laser therapy, or topical depigmenting agents, depending on the case.

The Four Horsemen of Pigmentation for Melanin-Rich Skin

If you're seeing changes to the skin and the skin's natural melanin that aren't genetic, it might be that external factors are coming into play. These can compromise skin, affect color and tone or damage the skin for good.

Some of the factors that can potentially damage or affect melanin in the skin include:

UV Radiation

Prolonged exposure to ultraviolet (UV) rays from the sun or artificial sources, like tanning beds, can damage melanocytes and alter melanin production. This damage can lead to irregular pigment distribution, causing issues like sunburn (aka Epithelial Cellular Apoptosis), tanning, or uneven pigmentation.

Harsh Chemical Exposure

Certain chemicals, like those in some skincare products or cosmetics, can interfere with melanin production or cause skin irritation, leading to pigmentation changes or damage to melanocytes. There are also Skin Bleaching Agents (SBA) to consider, which can be an incredibly damaging problem in some Melanin-Rich communities.

Inflammation and Skin Trauma

Injuries, acne, or skin conditions that cause inflammation can sometimes affect melanocytes, leading to changes in melanin production. Conditions like post-inflammatory hyperpigmentation (PIH) can result from this.

Hormonal Changes

Fluctuations in hormone levels, particularly during pregnancy or with hormonal treatments, can impact melanin production, leading to conditions like melasma (often referred to as the "mask of pregnancy").

If your client (of any gender) is experiencing these changes (or perhaps you are the client), a professional consultation with a Skin or Medical professional for support, advice and diagnosis is always the right step.

5

STEP INTO THE (MELANIN-RICH) CLASSROOM

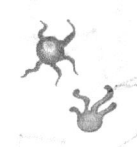

If you don't learn, and you're not open to new ideas, you're not going to develop as a Skin Pro...

In this chapter, you'll discover:

- The importance of education when it comes to CQ
- Skin concerns and conditions that you may not be as familiar with when it comes to Melanin-Rich skin
- How to have supportive conversations, rooted in CQ, with your clients

Diverse skin types and tones necessitate an understanding of variations in skin care needs. A culturally intelligent approach in skincare fosters inclusivity, recognizes global market diversity and allows brands to create products that resonate with Skin Pros and consumers of various cultural backgrounds.

WHY CQ ED IS KEY

When it comes down to understanding and being able to treat every shade of skin, as well as exhibiting genuine cultural intelligence (CQ), education is one of the most important pillars. If not *the* most important.

If you don't learn, and you're not open to new ideas, opinions and thought processes then you're not going to develop as a Skin Pro or an expert.

Things are improving. I'm seeing much more of a move towards education that is truly inclusive with governing bodies now including mandatory units on working with Melanin-Rich skin and textured hair. However, there are still many resources that don't cover a balanced view of working with Melanin-Rich skin. And I do mean *balanced*.

Historically, dermatology textbooks have featured Melanin-Rich skin in a biased way, or they've completely excluded it from the narrative unless it's been in a negative way. There are currently projects in place to shift this imbalance and bring dermatology resources into present times. Education fundamentals should embed skin that is Melanin-Rich as foundational to cease the "othering".

There's an ongoing project around decolonizing global health resources, led by Global Health Research Policy[1], focusing on making widely available health resources more accessible to everyone.

The Inclusive Skin Color Project[2] is a joint effort between the University of California San Francisco's School of Medicine's Anti-Oppression Curriculum (AOC) Initiative, the USCF Library and the Department of Dermatology. It aims to increase access to representative and inclusive images of skin findings to support representative teaching.

The University of Alberta[3] funded research to make strategic changes to their dermatology courses to include more representation of Melanin-Rich skin tones in their teaching materials to educate their students - the world's future dermatologists.

These are just a few projects that are going on right now. I know I'm not alone when I say, I'm *here* for it.

SKIN THEOLOGIAN'S SKINSIGHT

Early 2024, I released a social media skin health video series that focused on some of the things that may not be covered in conventional settings.

The goal was and always is to help Skin Pros and Clients alike to love their Melanin more, by UNDERSTANDING it. Yes, understanding dispels misuse & abuse.

Indifferent of your skin tone or background, fundamental, even bite-size, educational segments only help to diffuse the fear, or misconceptions around caring for skin of color.

Here are a few from that series:

- Inflammation 101 - Basics on making sure the first line of defense is up to keep undue hyper-pigmentation at bay.

- Cosmeceutical Vs. Cosmetic 101 - Avoid popularized comedogenic formulas on the skin, which don't serve the skin's health.

- Tyrosinase-Inhibitors Vs. Skin Bleaching Agents - what you need to know to make an informed and educated decision for skin health.

- STOP Using Petroleum Jelly on Your Skin as Skin Care - One of the most popular products that many cultures have grown up using, (believe me, I know, as I did), especially within Melanin-Rich skin communities: Using Petroleum Jelly. (Sorry but not sorry to all those obsessed with the 'slugging' trend).

Time to turn things up! Let's step into the Melanin-Rich classroom to level up the parts of working with Melanin-Rich skin that often go unaddressed and undervalued in traditional industry education pathways.

MELANIN-RICH: FUNDAMENTALS

Let's start with the fundamentals. Those need-to-knows that are often missing or overlooked when it comes to skincare education. This information is *essential*. It should never, ever be optional if you're going to be working with all skin types and tones - and especially if you're going to be working on Melanin-Rich skin, which you absolutely should be.

Class is in session, so gather around for the basics that you may not have seen covered in your educational programs (that definitely *should have* been there).

The first thing you need to know is that Hyperpigmentation is the primary concern in skin that is Melanin-Rich. Whether it is age-related, hormonal, acne, sun-induced or any other inflammatory-related trigger, hyperpigmentation is considered the secondary lesion as a result of the unresolved primary lesion: inflammation.

We need to know how to provide Hyperpigmentation treatments, safely. And that must include the use of anti-inflammatories.

Sometimes the solutions for hyperpigmentation that are discussed in mainstream educational resources are far from ideal for darker skin tones.

Melanin-Rich skin is more prone to hyperpigmentation. We discussed it in the last chapter. It's a common skin concern where patches of skin become darker in color than the surrounding areas. This occurs due to an excess production of melanin.

We need to be aware of two types of melanin that everyone produces in their skin: Eumelanin or Pheomelanin.

Remember, in darker skin tones, Eumelanin is the quality of pigment that is produced, and when hyperpigmentation occurs, it can show up as brownish-black spots within the skin.

In lighter skin tones, Pheomelanin is the quality of pigment that is produced, and when hyperpigmentation occurs, it can show up as reddish, purplish or even gray spots within the skin. [See Fig. 7.]

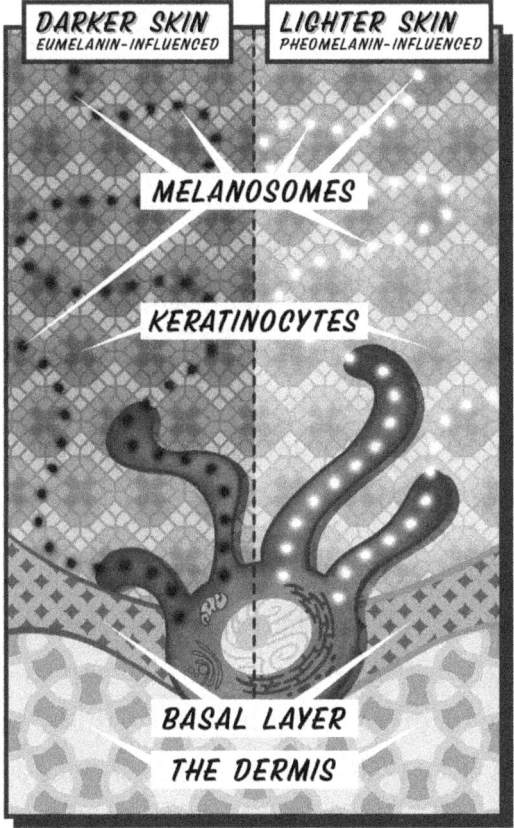

[Fig. 7.]

What we need to know is that Pheomelanin's property is naturally soluble, whereas Eumelanin (which influences darker skin tones) is less soluble. Solubility is paramount in the efficacious deliverability of active ingredients. In other words, it naturally takes longer for Melanin-Rich skin to be treated with formulas and treatment approaches, due to the nature of insolubility it possesses.

Don't get me wrong, both are treatable. One just takes longer.

You might see recommendations for topical treatments like Hydroquinone, Kojic Acid, Azelaic Acid, Retinoids or Vitamin C. Or you may see other physical treatments like microdermabrasion, micro-needling, (melanin-rich friendly) laser treatments and chemical peels recommended.

These *can* all be effective treatments but some can also cause more problems than they solve. Some of these treatments - for example, Microdermabrasion that is performed incorrectly or in a way that's too heavy-handed, as it's a technique-sensitive service - can cause inflammation, which leads to Post-Inflammatory Hyperpigmentation (PIH) in Melanin-Rich skin - this means more dark spots and a cycle of worry. Microneedling at too long a needle depth or if Acne is too far an aggressive grade but still microneedled, can also have adverse effects. In extreme, uncontrolled cases, it can even cause hypo-pigmentation. Now, that is certainly a level of damage we do not want to see.

Treatments for hyperpigmentation should always be used appropriately, and it's important to take the type and severity of the hyperpigmentation into account before just delving in with the strongest solution that's available.

It's also essential to recommend Pre-care before delivering a Professional service, as well as Post-care and use percentages of actives that are safe for Melanin-Rich skin.

This is even something to consider when it comes to treating breakouts and ongoing Acne. Acne treatments might vary for darker skin tones due to the risk of PIH or keloid scarring. Specialized education on effective Acne treatments without causing pigmentation issues is crucial.

Some inflammation isn't always visible to the naked eye, but it can still cause hyperpigmentation and damage to the skin. We'll talk about this in more detail as we go, but what are the main points you need to know about Melanin-Rich skin, acne, inflammation and hyperpigmentation? Here we go:

- According to research[4] clients who have Acne and Melanin-Rich skin are predisposed to greater levels of inflammation within the skin.
- Clients with Melanin-Rich skin and Acne have increased inflammatory processes involved in early levels of Acne formation.

- This type of inflammation is referred to as 'Subclinical' because it occurs before the Acne is visible.
- This is referred to as "persistent" inflammation rather than just "post-inflammation".
- I call this invisible inflammation. This likely helps us understand, at least in part, why PIH in deeper skin tones takes longer time to treat than within skin that is lighter in skin tones.

Next up is an age-old favorite (or not-so-favorite, as the misinformation around this can quite literally cost lives). There's a misconception that people with Melanin-Rich skin don't need sun protection.

Conventional education often neglects the importance of sunscreen and sun protection measures, leading to inadequate information about sun damage risks for darker skin and the necessity of protection.

As we've covered, all skin tones can experience skin damage and the risks associated with overexposure to UV rays. You need to know this fundamentally, and so do your clients: everyone needs to wear SPF daily. Even if it isn't sunny. Even if their skin is rich in beautiful melanin.

MELANIN-RICH: INTERMEDIARY

Here's a topic that I never see discussed enough when it comes to skin that is Melanin-Rich. And it can have some serious consequences for the skin. That topic is hidden or invisible erythema.

Because this is such an important topic not discussed enough when it comes to Melanin-Rich skin, I'm going to lay this study down again for the Intermediate Level of this chapter.

Erythema is redness of the skin, usually caused by inflammation, irritation, skin disorders, trauma, allergic reactions or infections. It can also be caused by some health conditions or medication side effects.

Anyone can experience erythema - you've probably experienced it yourself or seen it in your clients. It can vary in intensity, distribution, and duration depending on the underlying cause. Side note: it's essential that if you spot erythema in your client you identify the cause.

Your consultation process should help you rule out health conditions and medications, but it might be necessary to reiterate this with your client as sometimes they get so used to their daily routine or forget to mention relevant information.

Invisible or *hidden* erythema refers to the redness of the skin that might not be immediately visible to the naked eye, especially on Melanin-Rich skin where it's less easy to spot. This phenomenon can be a challenge for Skin Pros, and we must be aware of it for several reasons:

- **Risk of over-treatment** - if you can't visually detect erythema, there's a risk of over-treating the skin. Without the commonly taught apparent signs of inflammation, they might assume the skin can handle more aggressive treatments, leading to potential damage or complications.
- **Inaccurate assessment of skin health** - invisible erythema might mask underlying skin issues or reactions. Without proper recognition, Skin Pros might misinterpret the skin's condition, leading to inappropriate recommendations or treatments.
- **Unequal treatment outcomes** - failure to recognize invisible erythema in darker skin tones can result in unequal treatment outcomes. Darker skin might react differently to various treatments, and without accounting for this invisible erythema, professionals might not tailor treatments effectively.

Understanding how inflammatory mediators (aka, cells involved in the inflammatory cascade, like PIH) along with melanocytes interact is so important in managing various skin conditions, especially those related to pigmentation disorders or inflammatory skin diseases. Targeting these mediators or their pathways can potentially lead to the development of therapies aimed at controlling pigmentation disorders or inflammatory skin conditions.

SKIN THEOLOGIAN'S SKINSIGHT

Let's dig deep into some science for a second (which is what makes up the basis of the entire industry when you look at it) and talk about the Melanocyte-Langerhan cell connection.

This connection refers to the relationship between Dendrites (remember them?). Melanocytes and Langerhans cells, two of the dendritic and immune cells found in the epidermis. While they serve different functions, these two types of cells interact and collaborate in a few different ways within the skin's microenvironment.

Studies [5]suggest a possible interaction where Langerhans cells might influence Melanocyte function, particularly in the transfer of melanin. Some research shows that Langerhans cells can interact with neighboring melanocytes and affect pigmentation processes. [See Fig. 8]

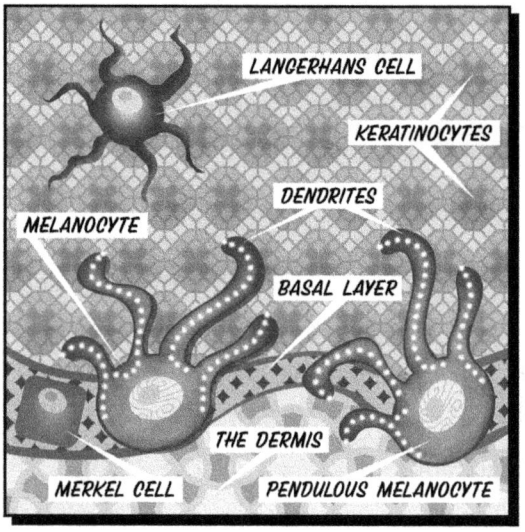

[Fig. 8.]

As you can see in this diagram, the environment of the Epidermis involves three specific Dendritic cells. The Langerhans cell, the Merkel cell and the Melanocyte cell. Studies are still emerging concerning new findings of all of these familial cells.

(Btw - there is yet another Dendritic cell that lives in the Dermis rather than the Epidermis. You and I know this to be called the Macrophage cell or White Blood Cell (WBC). Its role is Phagocytic, meaning it's a scavenger and eats up rebel invaders in the skin and body. And so, there you can see immune responses of these dendritic cells should not be so foreign to us.

Both cell types contribute to the skin's defense mechanisms too. Melanocytes produce melanin, which helps protect against UV radiation by absorbing and dissipating harmful rays. Langerhans cells, as part of the immune system, play a role in identifying and responding to potential threats in the skin.

Disruptions in the interaction between Melanocyte and Langerhans cells could contribute to various skin conditions, including pigmentary disorders or immune-mediated skin diseases.

Research into the precise nature of the connection between these two cell types is ongoing. Understanding their non-identical twin interaction could offer insights into skin health, immunity, and pigmentation disorders, as well as potentially lead to the development of therapies targeting skin conditions involving pigmentation. This is real progress.

And I know I'm not the only one who gets excited about it.

To address these challenges, Skin Pros should be trained to look for more subtle signs of inflammation or irritation beyond visible redness. This might involve considering other indicators such as warmth, texture changes or subjective feedback from the client, especially those with Melanin-Rich skin. They should also consider using imaging technologies or specialized tools that can detect skin changes beyond what's visible to the naked eye.

Let's also talk about lasers. You know we had to. You might not be aware that some types of lasers shouldn't be used on Melanin-Rich skin, or conversely, you may have been told that lasers are a no-no for Melanin-Rich skin altogether. Both of these assumptions are incorrect.

Laser treatments for Melanin-Rich skin require specific considerations due to the higher risk of complications such as post-inflammatory hyperpigmentation (PIH), hypopigmentation, or scarring. The main concern lies in the laser's ability to target the chromophore; melanin, as darker skin has higher melanin concentrations as we covered earlier, making it more prone to absorbing excessive laser energy, potentially leading to damage.

Essentially, *Selective PhotoThermolysis* is what we are talking about. The destruction of certain chromophores that are selected by the laser beam heat. Melanin (pigment), Hemoglobin (vascular) and Water (collagen-stimulating) all contain chromophores that laser energy is attracted to. Laser stands for '***Light Amplification by the Stimulated Emission of Radiation***'. Some wavelengths are off-limits to skin that is more chromophore-heavy.

Lasers with shorter wavelengths, like some types of CO_2 or certain types of IPL (Intense Pulsed Light), have a higher risk of causing pigmentation changes or burns in darker skin tones due to their greater absorption by melanin, and greater delivery of energy.

Ablative lasers, like some CO_2 or erbium-based lasers, remove layers of skin. While effective for certain issues, they pose a higher risk of post-inflammatory hyperpigmentation and scarring in darker skin due to their intensity.

Longer wavelengths penetrate deeper, bypassing the epidermal melanin. The energy is less and therefore, the risk of heating the epidermis and causing unnecessary damage to the skin.

The laser's ability to target specific chromophores (like melanin) without causing collateral damage to surrounding tissue is crucial. Pulse duration, energy levels, and cooling methods used during the treatment influence the risk of adverse effects.

The experience of the practitioner using the laser is essential too. I call these technique-sensitive treatments. If you haven't had full training in lasers or don't feel like you're confident and understand what you're doing, please don't go there. It might seem straightforward, but there's a reason that there's usually specific training on lasers just for Skin Pros.

An experienced Skin Pro understands how to adjust settings and choose the right laser for darker skin safely. If you offer laser treatments, you need to understand how to use them safely for every single shade and type of skin.

Laser treatments for dark skin require a cautious approach and often necessitate a longer recovery period. Pre-treatment measures such as skin conditioning, (sometimes) using bleaching agents, or avoiding sun exposure are crucial to minimize risks.

So, which lasers are generally safe for Melanin-Rich skin? I'll start by saying to make sure you seek guidance from your laser provider or trainer on the specific device brand you're using - I can provide general education between these pages, but sometimes you need to do a little extra homework, especially on such an important topic. Here's the current list of lasers (at the time of publishing) that are considered "safe" when it comes to Melanin-Rich skin:

- **Nd:YAG Lasers** - these lasers have longer wavelengths that can penetrate deeper into the skin while minimizing melanin absorption. They're safer for darker skin tones as they reduce the risk of pigmentation changes or burns.
- **Fractional Lasers** - fractional lasers create microscopic treatment zones, sparing surrounding tissue. Fractional devices like fractional non-ablative lasers or fractionated erbium lasers are safer for dark skin.
- **Q-Switched Lasers** - specifically, Q-switched Nd:YAG lasers can effectively target pigmented lesions while minimizing damage to the surrounding skin.
- **Pico Laser** - This is one of the newest and increasingly popularized types of lasers out in the market (at the time of publication). It is considered safe for all skin including Fitzpatrick 4,5 and 6.

When you understand the physiology of the skin, the realm of the laser device and its technique delivery, you remove the fear equation.

MELANIN-RICH: ADVANCED LEVEL

Skin bleaching is - unfortunately - more common than you may think in some communities. And if it isn't something that you've seen or felt familiar with before, then you may not recognize it (at least not immediately).

It involves the use of chemicals or substances to lighten the skin tone. It's typically done to achieve a lighter complexion, and it isn't usually done safely, carefully or without compromising the skin on some level.

Prolonged use of these chemicals can lead to serious health issues, including skin irritation, allergic reactions, thinning of the skin, acne, stretch marks, and even long-term complications like kidney damage, neurological problems, or increased risk of skin cancer.

Often driven by societal pressures or cultural beliefs associated with lighter skin tones, skin bleaching can have significant psychological effects as well as physical effects too, leading to low self-esteem, body image issues, and mental health concerns.

As a Skin Pro, recognizing signs of skin bleaching is crucial to providing appropriate guidance and care.

In addition, it is extremely *(emphasis added)* important to approach all clients with Cultural Intelligence. Insensitive and shaming approaches have never and will never support client awareness. I would be remiss if I didn't state that under a Physician's care, some Skin Bleaching Agents (SBA) have yielded good results.

But these Physician-led approaches should only be temporary, and should never be prolonged. The truth is, there's a vista of reasons why people resort to (SBAs). Leading with judgment will never serve anyone well. Take the time to hear their story and support them accordingly.

Here are some signs you may want to watch out for:

- **Uneven skin tone** - look for irregular or uneven skin lightening that doesn't appear natural. Bleaching can result in patches of significantly lighter skin amidst the natural skin tone. You may also notice an unnaturally flat, dull-looking skin with no natural sheen.
- **Abrupt color changes** - Be cautious of sudden changes in skin color or dramatic lightening in specific areas of the skin, especially when it doesn't correspond to typical responses from skincare treatments.
- **Skin texture changes** - bleaching agents might cause changes in skin texture, such as thinning, increased sensitivity, or a glossy appearance.

- **Excessive sensitivity to sun** - skin that has undergone bleaching is extremely sensitive to sunlight, leading to rapid sunburns or increased skin reactions upon sun exposure.
- **Presence of side effects** - be alert for signs of skin irritation, redness, or inflammation in areas where bleaching agents might have been applied.

Approaching this topic, or discussing it with your clients can be a challenge. It's a sensitive matter (in more ways than one) and comes with significant societal and cultural considerations.

First, you need to create a supportive and trusting environment between you and your client. Ensure the client feels comfortable and safe during the conversation. Try these **CQ Tips:** Use a warm, non-judgmental tone and convey that your goal is to understand their skincare concerns fully.

Begin by expressing your concern for their skin health. You might say:

SAMPLE: "I've noticed some changes in your skin tone, and my priority is ensuring the health and well-being of your skin. Have you recently made any changes to your skincare routine or used specific products?"

Refrain from making assumptions about their skincare practices. Instead, focus on observing changes in their skin and gently inquire about any factors that might have contributed to those changes.

Emphasize your willingness to listen and support them. You could say:

SAMPLE: "I understand that skincare concerns can be personal, and I'm here to help. If there's anything you'd like to discuss or any specific concerns you have, I'm here to assist you."

If the client confirms using skin-lightening products, approach the conversation with empathy and educate them about potential risks sensitively. Emphasize your commitment to their skin's health and suggest alternative skincare approaches that focus on promoting a healthy complexion without resorting to harmful practices.

Enjoying what you've read so far?
Leave Us A Review on the site where you made this purchase.
It Helps To Spread Skin Health Equity Through Literature

6

MELANIN-RICH: PRO PERSPECTIVES

ULTIMATE FORMATTING - SAVE FOR QR CODE AND LINK

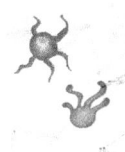

They speak to clients and students daily...

I n this chapter, you'll see:

- What Skin Pros really think about the industry, CQ and the conversation around Melanin-Rich skin
- Where the opportunities for improvement sit within the industry

A SKIN PRO'S PERSPECTIVE

One of the perspectives that I wanted to bring you in this book was the perspective of the Skin Professional, other than my own. These skilled and informed Skin Professionals come from a diverse set of backgrounds, experiences and life stages.

They speak to clients and students daily, and hear first-hand what they think, say and do when it comes to their experiences.

Many of these Experts have seen big changes in the industry over time too, and I felt that it was incredibly important to reflect on their insights and knowledge.

I interviewed six Skin Pros, working in different parts of the industry, for a variety of brands (or themselves), some as Educators to seasoned and new and upcoming Skin Professionals. It was important for me to have international representation, and I was honored to reach out to some of the best, I know in the skin space. Here's what they had to say about what the professional skin space looks like when it comes to Melanin-Rich Skin.

"What is your perspective on the landscape of the Professional Skin industry concerning Melanin-Rich skin over the recent years or throughout your tenure in the field? Please elaborate on the motivations behind your work and its impact on addressing the specific needs of Melanin-Rich skin?"

"Over the years, I've witnessed a positive shift in acknowledging and catering to Melanin-Rich Skin in the skincare industry. There have been expanded product lines, more diversity in advertising and more educational initiatives being offered by institutions and organizations.

I do what I do in order to rectify historically neglected and underrepresentation of diverse skin tones. I aim to bridge the gap by advocating for inclusive skin care practices, ensuring all skin types receive proper care and attention."

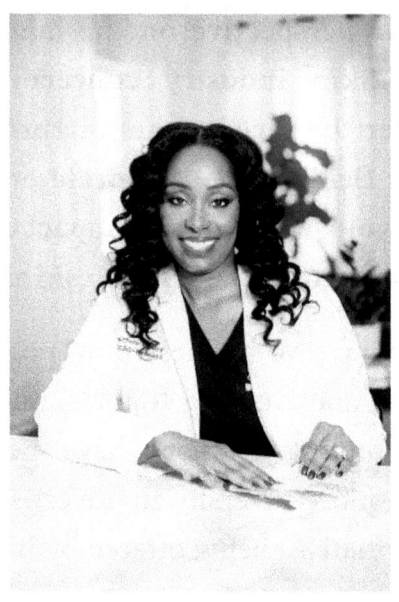

Nichelle Mosley, North Carolina + California
Award Winning, Corneotherapist Trainer,
Educator, CEO & Founder
The Skin Barrier Academy
Managing Director for Fearless Beauties

"My aesthetics career started in 2017, and shortly after entering the field and hearing skin horror stories from clients of color, I knew my space within the industry would be focused on clients with Melanin-Rich skin. I felt like most spas/skin professionals didn't care or see the need to educate themselves on a population that makes up most of the Greater Toronto area."

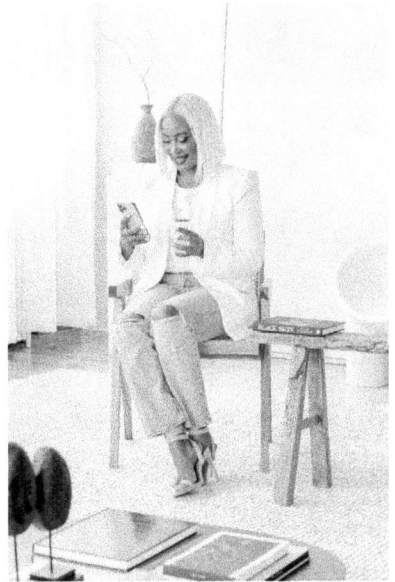

Orica Smart, Toronto
Award Winning Multicultural Skin Care Therapist

"I've been in the beauty industry for the past 6 years and a licensed esthetician for the past 3 years and there have been positive changes concerning Melanin-Rich skin. There are more options and resources available than there were even just 10 years ago.

As a Black man, when I get a first-time client that has Melanin-Rich skin I see a sigh of relief and they tell me they instantly feel more comfortable. Only about 5% of licensed estheticians are Black so I believe my purpose is to take up as much space as I can in the skin-care/beauty industry to make it easier for others."

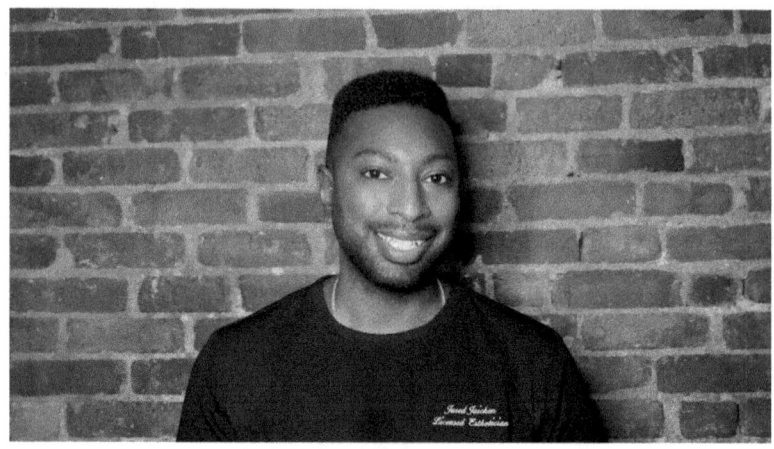

Jared Jaichon, New Jersey
Licenced Esthetician and Dermalogica Expert

"When I graduated I got my first job as a Skin Therapist working in a clinic with about 95% Fitzpatrick 1-2 performing a lot of Skin Peels and I distinctly remember there were approximately 5 clients who had aboriginal, Asian and Hispanic ancestry with what I would define now as Fitzpatrick 4 and 5 and when I performed the same peel treatment on their skin it did not respond the same as Fitzpatrick 1 and 2 clients.

Quite often the hyperpigmentation they were treating would appear darker and the skin would experience more sensation and heat during the service. Had I been trained initially with understanding the best treatment choices, processing times and aftercare these clients would have had more effective treatment outcomes."

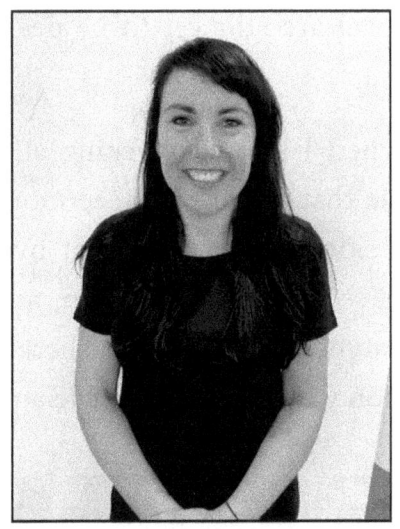

Susan Neilon, Brisbane
Skin Health & Dermal Institute Educator

"Being in the skincare industry for nearly 25 years, you can imagine how much I've seen it evolve with treatments, technology and gold standard ingredients and I believe we are only just scratching the surface of this topic. Consumers are a lot more savvy these days with the vast array of information that can be found on the internet, however, there's still a massive hole in the industry as a way of education for both consumers and Skin Pros. There are increasing amounts of treatments available for Melanin-Rich skin, but the more advanced treatments that target concerns such as pigmentation and hair removal are still yet to be deemed 'safe and effective'.

It was only when I started working at a doctor and nurse-led clinic that I started to see more clients with Melanin-Rich skin. I would say that over half of my clients now have Melanin-Rich skin, and the biggest concern I treat is pigmentation. There's definitely a lack of education when it comes to Melanin-Rich skin."

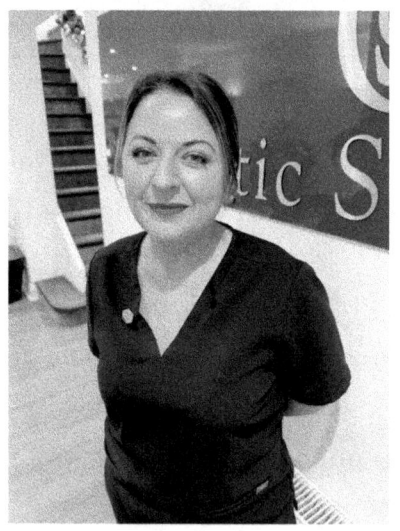

Amanda Matcham, UK
Skin Specialist, The Cosmetic Skin Clinic

"In my 23 years of practice in this industry, it's unfortunate to say that it has not always been easy connecting with information that is related to Melanin-Rich skin.

Fast forward, to today, things have certainly changed, and we are seeing more information and knowledge being shared. Being an educator for the past decade has truly opened up my horizons in realizing that I have to be the voice of educating people on Melanin-Rich skin.

I remember feeling uncomfortable talking about Melanin-Rich skin to a class filled with colleagues who did not have Melanin-Rich skin. It was only after a while, that I met people who also believed in the importance of educating all skin types and tones that I realized that it was up to me to continue to teach others and my students who were

becoming professionals in learning and also respecting all skin types. Leading by example had to start with me but the average skin professional - including dermatologists - are not confident in diagnosing or treating Melanin-Rich skin. I do what I do because the skincare industry has long failed to consider and reflect the needs of darker skin tones."

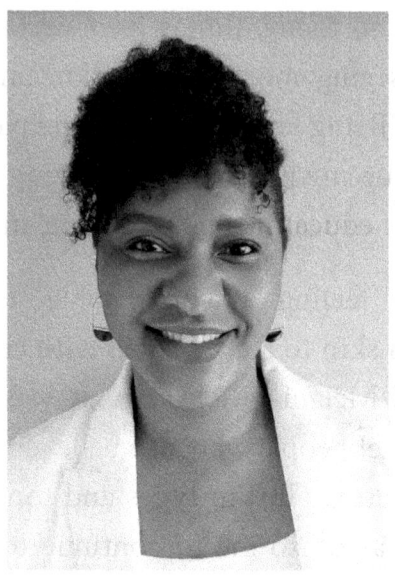

Magdalene Lafontant, Canada
Skin Academy Educator Founder and CEO of PEMA Canada

"In your professional expertise, what hurdles have Skin Professionals encountered in caring for, understanding, learning about, or administering treatments for Melanin-Rich Skin within a professional setting?"

"I think the limited education and training on diverse skin types are significant hurdles for Skin Pros. There's also an inadequate curriculum and limited access to resources - as a result, professionals may graduate without sufficient knowledge, hands-on experience or opportunities to enhance their knowledge. There's also complexity in skin diversity, which continues to enhance the need for a comprehensive educational path. This has the potential to have a huge impact on client care."

> **Nichelle Mosley, North Carolina + California**
> **Award Winning, Corneotherapist Trainer,**
> **Educator, CEO & Founder**
> **The Skin Barrier Academy**
> **Managing Director for Fearless Beauties**

"The main hurdle would be education. Taking the extra steps necessary to educate yourself and your team on the practical skin procedures and products, as well as education on race and unconscious biases, are needed too. Darker skin tones can suffer from biases and misconceptions in the skin space - it doesn't feel like there are enough courses in Canada that cover these things."

> **Orica Smart, Toronto**
> **Award-Winning Multicultural Skin Care Therapist**

"In most beauty schools there's still only one chapter or small section focused on treating Melanin-Rich skin. It feels like the excuse is, because we have Melanin-Rich skin we don't have to care for it and we don't have to do as much, when that is simply not true. The majority of what I learned about Melanin-Rich skin was outside of school, through trial and error on my own skin and researching articles and books."

Jared Jaichon, New Jersey
Licenced Esthetician and Dermalogica Expert

"The primary hurdle is still a lack of education when treating Melanin-Rich skin. Some skin education and device companies are doing very well in this space however there is a long way to go in other colleges and training spaces. I see this demonstrated when training skin therapists who feel at a loss and, to be honest, afraid to treat clients who have Melanin-Rich skin. They would rather not treat their skin as they don't know the safe parameters.

Recently, two of my colleagues and I enrolled in Dermal Therapies Training after attaining our Diplomas in Beauty Therapy many years ago. I have been heartened to see the inclusion of Melanin-Rich skin treatment references to provide safe and effective treatment outcomes."

Susan Neilon, Brisbane
Skin Health & Dermal Institute Educator

"In my professional opinion, a hurdle for me starts from the beginning. EDUCATION. I still feel like there's a stigma on who will be better equipped to help with Melanin-Rich skin concerns. The language that you use and where you live in the world has shown me just how different people can be."

Amanda Matcham, UK
Skin Specialist, The Cosmetic Skin Clinic

"I have noticed and observed that our textbooks fail us. Everything starts with a foundation, which should start with the schools. When you open an esthetics textbook, there is hardly a topic on multicultural skin types. There is a huge lack of education on this matter. The primary hurdle has been Hyperpigmentation.

This is one of the hardest hurdles for both new and seasoned professionals, Skin Professionals relying on the Fitzpatrick scale have inaccurate indicators when it comes to predicting sun sensitivities. Most of the books exposed to the new and seasoned Skin Professionals lack information on how some of these scales affect Melanin-Rich skin when it comes to treating hyperpigmentation and using chemical peels or laser treatments."

Magdalene Lafontant, Canada

Skin Academy Educator Founder and CEO of PEMA
Canada

"In your professional viewpoint, what are the foremost challenges faced by consumers and clients in adopting healthy skin care practices tailored for Melanin-Rich skin?"

"Clients often face challenges in finding suitable skincare products that address their specific needs.

Misinformation from social media and influencers as well as lack of tailored guidance contribute to confusion in establishing effective skincare routines too. Clients also don't always have the confidence in seeking appropriate skincare advice."

Nichelle Mosley, North Carolina + California
Award Winning, Corneotherapist Trainer,
Educator, CEO & Founder
The Skin Barrier Academy
Managing Director for Fearless Beauties

"Some top hurdles for consumers would be education on how their skin operates, the importance of sunscreen and access to Skin Pros who are equipped to treat their skin concerns with confidence."

Orica Smart, Toronto
Award-Winning Multicultural Skin Care Therapist

"When consumers don't see themselves represented by a brand it can feel as if they don't exist or that brand just isn't for them. Most consumers give up after trying multiple products and spending their hard-earned money that ultimately doesn't work for their skin and end up feeling defeated."

Jared Jaichon, New Jersey
Licenced Esthetician and Dermalogica Expert

"The top hurdle for consumers is understanding safe treatment and self-care for their own skin. No matter what the Fitzpatrick classification a consumer presents, they can be swayed very easily toward what their favorite influencer loves or uses on their skin. Being uneducated and unaware of the nuances of their own skin and its compatibility with the desired product or treatment, they may make a risky choice and unknowingly damage their skin in the process. Education for clients is the first step and this should be from the provider of the product or device, perhaps even a warning label or processing time variance, this may be the way forward."

Susan Neilon, Brisbane
Skin Health & Dermal Institute Educator

"I think the biggest hurdle is getting their head around the fact that ALL skin types need SPF. I find this the hardest to drill into my patients so again I educate them. The problem is finding a decent SPF that doesn't have a chalky finish. I also think that a lot of skincare companies, social media platforms and general advertising are generally based around Caucasian skin. Even companies that offer tinted products, only cater to lighter skin tones. In 25 years I've never worked alongside a company that offers this. As the second largest industry in the world, this is shocking!"

Amanda Matcham, UK
Skin Specialist, The Cosmetic Skin Clinic

"The definition of beauty has always been very Western-centric, which has led to a skincare industry that has long failed to consider and reflect the needs of all skin. There are too many myths and misconceptions - these need to be solved by education.

Melanin-Rich skin is - incorrectly - considered as 'tough' because this is what society has made us believe. We have come a long way when it comes to information and products. We need to support all clients in getting what they need."

Magdalene Lafontant, Canada
Skin Academy Educator Founder and CEO of PEMA
Canada

"Over the last five years, how would you characterize the progress in the Professional Skin Health sector concerning the availability of resources, courses, materials, and representation specifically tailored for Melanin-Rich Skin? Would you categorize the improvement as (0-mild), (mild-moderate), or (moderate–exceptional)? Kindly provide insights into your perspective on why this progression has occurred."

"There has been progress when it comes to resources and representation, with increased awareness and advocacy - but there's still plenty of room for growth. Education on Melanin-Rich skin needs to come as standard and be accessible."

Nichelle Mosley, North Carolina + California
Award Winning, Corneotherapist Trainer,
Educator, CEO & Founder
The Skin Barrier Academy
Managing Director for Fearless Beauties

"I would say the space has mildly improved. Clients with Melanin-Rich skin have become more vocal in their wants and needs, and this is being reflected in brand marketing. I do wonder how much this translates to actual client experience, however."

Orica Smart, Toronto
Award Winning Multicultural Skin Care Therapist

"Through the power of social media there has been a mild to moderate improvement for available melanin-rich skin resources especially after the summer of 2020 with the BLM movement. It forced everyone to have those difficult conversations about inclusivity and how companies could be doing more."

Jared Jaichon, New Jersey
Licenced Esthetician and Dermalogica Expert

"In the past 5 years I would say that there has been a mild increase in the provision of training in Melanin Rich Skin. I see this in the number of therapists I train at the organization I work for. I do feel however the therapists need to revise and revisit this training to keep it at the forefront of their mind."

Susan Neilon, Brisbane

Skin Health & Dermal Institute Educator

"Honestly – I think the change has been extremely mild and going back to how far we have come with treatments, technology and ingredients, it's the ingredients that are making the most impact. The research and development of such fabulous products ARE what can really make a difference to someone's skin and any good therapist should know this. In terms of materials and resources made available.

Any consumer or therapist out there must….educate, educate, educate."

Amanda Matcham, UK
Skin Specialist, The Cosmetic Skin Clinic

"I would say the professional skin health space has seen moderate to exceptional improvement. There has been an ever-growing crop of skincare brands coming to the market in the past five years that have been specifically formulated for skin of color. There have also been a lot of professional organizations that have been managing to connect other professionals with education in this regard.

There has also been more education and awareness about the role of Melanin-Rich skin and how to care for it properly. Thanks to professionals who have been pushing companies to enlighten new and seasoned professionals, they have been launching a lot of online courses for skin therapists and future professionals to help strengthen their knowledge in this regard. A lot of professionals are also recognizing the gap that has been missed for far too long."

Magdalene Lafontant, Canada
Skin Academy Educator Founder and CEO of PEMA
Canada

SKIN THEOLOGIAN'S SKINSIGHT

There's a clear thread that runs through every single set of insights from these experienced and knowledgeable Skin Pros: EDUCATION.

Whether it's standard beauty education pathways encompassing comprehensive training on working with clients with Melanin-Rich skin through to brands and client education also doing the same, this was consistently thought of as the biggest barrier for Skin Pros and consumers.

Many Skin Pros and clients have had to teach themselves and work out what's going to work for their skin through trial and error. This isn't good enough and shouldn't be acceptable. Especially when we have so much information available at the touch of a button nowadays. There's no reason why it can't be incorporated into educational programs right at the beginning, so that new Skin Pros can nail working with Melanin-Rich skin right from the get-go. It's important.

There's a general consensus that education has gotten a little better in recent years but we've still got a way to go to ensure that everyone understands Melanin-Rich skin and how to work with it.

It seems that there's also a perception that some of these changes don't go far enough - and that some may give the appearance of being inclusive but it's pretty surface-level. I don't think that that's wrong.

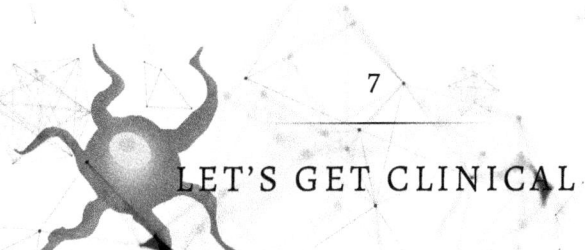
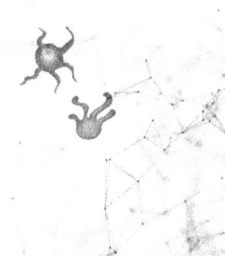

7

LET'S GET CLINICAL

The first step to understanding skin is to understand science.

In this chapter, you'll discover:

- How melanin presents in the skin
- The importance of representation on the clinical side of the industry
- Skin safety for clients

THE SCIENCE BEHIND SKIN

As a Skin Professional, our passion is what drives our growth. One of my passions as a Skin Pro | Author | Educator is for research-based findings, with every type of work I produce.

It is my professional opinion that clinical studies should be a part of every Skin Professional's arsenal in tandem with continual education, books, courses, articles, trade shows, conferences etc.

With the speed at which our industry evolves, we have to remain aware of the 'come and go trends', fictional and factual realities of the space.

The Immune Defence of the Melanocyte Cell

According to research[1] melanogenesis, the production of melanin, is suggested to be a by-product of enhanced immunity that doesn't have a clear function.

Melanin's roles in different species, including humans, are uncertain. It's widespread in both people and animals, evolving over 500 million years ago.

In mammals, melanin is part of an essential antimicrobial defense system. The process involves Tyrosinase as the initial enzyme, producing melanin that traps and kills microorganisms and exhibits antimicrobial activity. The precursors of melanin synthesis, L-tyrosine and L-dopa, show antiviral properties.

Melanocytes, originating from melanoblasts during the development of an embryo, remain consistent across different skin color populations.

Genetically, biochemically, and functionally, immunity and melanization are linked. Melanin may influence immunological responses too. Conditions causing albinism and impaired immunity further highlight this genetic connection.

This research suggests that certain disorders that affect the skin's pigmentation may have reduced antimicrobial defense.

Melanosomes, containing enzymes, act as barriers against disease-causing microorganisms. Normal human melanocytes contribute to the skin's immune defense system, in part due to its inherent immune function.

Skin, health and melanin are more interconnected than initially thought.

GENETICS AND MELANIN

If you've ever pondered the intricate relationship between genetics and pigmentary disorders, you're not alone.

I mentioned earlier in this work, the beautiful complexity of Melanin. An article in 'Experimental Dermatology' confirms the same, stating, 'Cutaneous pigmentation is an extremely complex human trait...'[2].

Human genes and gene mutations can be meticulously mapped out on cutaneous chromophores, primarily melanin.

These genetic pathways often lead to what dermatology textbooks term 'melanotic disorders', shedding light on the intricate interplay between genetics and skin pigmentation.

For those of you with a scientific curiosity, I encourage delving into these studies such as the one on hyper-melanotic and hypo-melanotic disorders in dermatology, footnoted in this chapter. I think you'll find invaluable genetic insights into the mechanisms underlying various melanin-related conditions.

With over 100 genes involved in the process of Melanogenesis, DNA encoding is critical. Any interruption to or intercellular trafficking of these messages between cells can affect Melanin synthesis.

The Importance of Diversity in Chemistry and Brand Production

The importance of diversity in chemistry and skincare brand production should never be understated. In-depth research [3] and analysis from CEW UK, The MBS Group and ScienceMagic.Inc. calls diversity in the beauty industry a "business critical issue." They also acknowledge that the industry is well-positioned for progress. I agree.

Diverse perspectives in chemistry lead to the development of skincare products that cater to a wide range of skin types, tones and concerns. Addressing diverse needs ensures that skincare products are effective and suitable for a broad consumer base.

Let's take a closer look at Sula Labs as an example. They're a collective of chemists, product development experts, and scientists passionate about dark skin and Black-owned brands.

Operating as a cosmetic R&D lab they develop and test formulas and ingredients for darker skin tones & Black-owned brands - including brands affiliated with Ulta Beauty, Sephora and Credo Beauty as well as indie brands.

They're led by a Black chemist and based in Los Angeles, California. They also share insights and research that relate to Melanin-Rich skin and beauty product development.

Sula Labs aims to bring chemistry transparency to the forefront for both brands and consumers. The small team based in California continues to garner clientele from all areas of beauty to ensure skincare regimens are tried and true, but most of all, safe to use on Melanin-Rich skin. The end goal is to expand its patent formulas and become the first laboratory to publish papers that dive into the morphological findings of Black complexions.

Diverse teams in brand production contribute to more accurate and respectful representation in marketing materials.

Consumers are more likely to connect with and trust brands that showcase diversity, as it reflects the reality of their customer base. Look at brands like Fenty Beauty and Black Girl Sunscreen who have put inclusivity at the center of what they do.

A representative team brings CQ to the production process, helping avoid insensitive marketing or formulation choices. It also fosters a rich exchange of ideas and perspectives, promoting innovation in skincare formulations and product development.

This approach also contributes to creative problem-solving and product development, a (potential) wider market reach, consumer empowerment and corporate social responsibility. It's all positive changes that can contribute to the next generation of Skin Pros.

SKIN THEOLOGIAN'S SKINSIGHT

In my industry interaction, I have the delight of meeting extraordinary professionals all the time. Recently, I connected with a Cosmetics Scientist and Product Formulator who specializes in formulating innovations with Melanin-Rich skin in mind.

Her craft and years of dedication have been centered around optimizing formulas that bear all of the nuances associated with Eumelanin-influenced pigment.

This is always encouraging to me, as an Author & Skin Health Equity Expert, as it takes "a village" to make a shift in the health and wellness space. With whom are you making connections within your space of business, skillset and career? We can all align with others of like passions for inspiration and greater awareness.

Dermal and Epidermal Hyperpigmentation

So, you read it earlier. Hyperpigmentation is a big deal, especially when it comes to Melanin-Rich skin. That's why you hear it mentioned so often - it's one of the top skin concerns that you'll hear mentioned from clients with darker skin tones and it's all linked to melanin, as we've discussed.

However, epidermal hyperpigmentation is more commonly discussed. I'm going to guess that you have always seen epidermal hyperpigmentation covered in educational sources rather than dermal. Sometimes, you have to let your passion shine through and dig a little deeper to find out the details that will make a difference to your clients and their skin.

Epidermal hyperpigmentation occurs in the epidermis, the outermost layer of the skin. It can be caused by sun exposure, inflammation, hormonal changes (like pregnancy) or injuries. Think of it as a surface-level pigmentation change.

Dermal hyperpigmentation occurs in the dermis, the deeper layer of the skin. It can be caused by long-term inflammation, PIH, medications and genetic factors. As previously discussed, the source is always the Melanocyte cell, but often, a pendulous one. [See earlier Fig.8.]

When it comes to epidermal hyperpigmentation, there are many treatments - it isn't a one-size-fits-all solution, unfortunately. However, these treatments are backed by research [4] and science. Dermal pigmentation is usually more difficult to reduce the visibility of, but with the right combination of treatments, it can be significantly improved.

Advanced, Non-Ablative lasers in combination with some staggering treatments such as superficial peels, in some cases, microneedling at a safe needle depth and other rejuvenating treatments.

Your CQ consultation is your standard bearer in determining epidermal from dermal pigmentary disorders.

8

STEP INTO THE TREATMENT ROOM

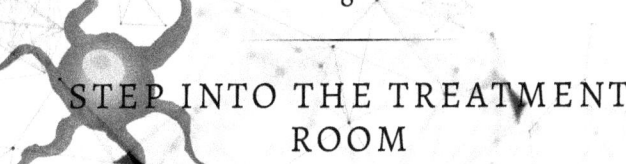

> *Although she doesn't exist as an individual, her experiences are all too real.*

In this chapter, you'll explore:

- Why it's so important to understand all of your clients
- What it's like to be Melanin-Rich and seeking a new Skin Pro

UNDERSTANDING YOUR CLIENTELE

If you're a Skin Pro, you might think that booking an appointment with you is easy, right?

Your appointment booking link is on your website and social media, your business is listed in all the right places and your phone number is front and center.

The social media feeds associated with your business are filled with client photos and information about your services - before and afters, testimonials, information about the products you use, new treatment launches, training you've been on, and the works.

Your booking process is clear, you're on hand to answer any questions within a reasonable amount of time and the directions to your space are right out there.

Should be straightforward, right? Even if you're not a professional in the industry, whenever you need to book a consultation or appointment it's all pretty easy to get to grips with, isn't it? You do a quick Google, browse some socials, take a look at prices, read some reviews, make an appointment and you're good to go.

Now let's put you in the shoes of a potential client with Melanin-Rich skin who's looking to find a new Skin Pro, make an appointment with them and have a stress-free experience where they leave with their skin rejuvenated and in great shape.

SETTING THE SCENE

We're going to start by setting the scene. The client perspective we're going to look at this scenario from is a 38-year-old woman with Melanin-Rich skin who lives in Canada. She's just moved to a new area and her tried-and-trusted beauty professionals are all now located too far away, in an area it's unlikely she'll be visiting regularly.

In her previously lived area, she had a hair stylist, nail technician and Skin Pro that she trusted unequivocally. She knew that they were great at what they did, comfortable with her skin and hair, consummate professionals, delivered great results every time, had great customer service, offered services that she wanted and their prices sat within her budget. This was after some trial and error, and many visits to beauty spaces that didn't work for her in the past.

Now, she has to begin the process of finding the right professionals for her needs, so we'll join her at the beginning of the process from her point of view. This will help you understand the real experience of people with Melanin-Rich skin and their experiences in the space.

This fictional client is made up of the lived experiences of the many women with Melanin-Rich skin that I know in both my personal and professional life. Although she doesn't exist as an individual, her experiences are all too real.

THE RESEARCH PHASE

It starts with the research phase. Just like anyone looking for an industry professional, she starts by asking for recommendations from friends and colleagues in her new area and starts searching online (including social media) to gather up her research.

Here's what she has to say about this part of the process:

"As someone with Melanin-Rich skin, finding the right skincare specialist can be a journey. I've learned that not all skincare treatments or products cater to my needs. So, when it comes to booking a beauty appointment, it's not just about finding any available slot; it's about finding a professional who understands the nuances of my skin.

There's a certain level of apprehension that comes with each booking. Will the specialist be knowledgeable about my skin? Will they have experience in dealing with hyperpigmentation? Are they going to damage my skin or tell me they don't know how to work with it? I know my friend tried a place like this and I *know* what she thought about it. If I ask too many questions are they going to decide I'm too much work as a client? Am I going to come out of here and head straight into somewhere else to fix what's happened?

Sometimes, it's frustrating to see a lack of representation too. The number of times I find someone who looks great, only to realize they have no clients that look like me appearing on their social media testimonials or they're using products that aren't good for my skin. Or I'll ask a question and they'll give me answers that I know mean they don't understand what's safe for my skin. Many ads show products and services that might not be suitable for me. It leaves me feeling unseen and overlooked.

But despite the challenges, I persevere. I actively seek out Skin Pro's who specialize in treating Melanin-Rich skin. They don't have to have Melanin-Rich skin themselves, but it's sometimes tougher to find someone who isn't and feels comfortable working with my skin.

Recommendations from other Melanin-Rich friends, family and colleagues or online communities become my guiding light. When I finally find someone who understands the needs of my skin, it's like discovering a hidden gem. I hold on to that Skin Pro for dear life and am faithful to a fault.

I'd describe the process as being pretty labor-intensive - it involves a mix of cautious optimism plus a desire to be understood and seen."

Ok, pause right there, my faithful Skin Pro reader, how does that sound to you?

On the one hand, you might think it doesn't sound too different from the process anyone has to undertake to find a new expert, but there are hidden challenges and nuances that people who don't have Melanin-Rich skin won't have to think about, such as:

1. Are the recommendations I'm getting from people who have a similar life experience or background to me?
2. Is the Skin Pro I'm looking at comfortable working with Melanin-Rich skin?
3. Are they experienced and knowledgeable about some of the differences between routines and products when it comes to Melanin-Rich skin?

4. Are they showing real results on people who look like me?
5. Do I need to worry that they're going to say or do anything that makes me feel uncomfortable about my skin?

Again…this is all actual feedback provided by clients with Melanin-Rich skin. Things they are thinking, that they might not feel confident or comfortable expressing to a Skin Professional.

GET THE BOOKING

Your prospective client has narrowed it down to three different specialists and sent a couple of questions to clarify if they're the right Skin Pro for her or on a couple of the treatments on offer.

She doesn't hear back from one of the Skin Professionals, which happens sometimes. Another Skin Pro replies with answers that demonstrate her understanding of all shades of skin is possibly not quite up to date. The third Skin Pro gets a gold star, answering promptly, professionally and in a way that shows she understands the skin she's (potentially) going to be working with.

That's who the client chooses to book with. But sometimes, especially in less diverse locations, there isn't even an option of one to choose from which can be a challenge. Or there's one person in the area who's the go-to for Melanin-Rich skin. That's a great position for the Skin Pro, but not always so great for the client.

THE FIRST APPOINTMENT

Heading to meet my new Skin Pro, I'm hopeful but a little nervous. I've had mixed experiences - some get my skin, others not so much. And when they don't, or worse when they pretend they do but I can tell they don't, it's frustrating. It shouldn't be this tough.

When I finally meet them, I do feel I have to be vigilant. But as we chat, I start feeling better. They listen and don't say anything that's a red flag.

They suggest a routine treatment that's tailored to my skin, not some generic plan. And they take time to explain why each step matters for me. I can see they know their product line as well as their service options back and front, and how it supports me.

I love it when it's like this but it does take some of the enjoyment and relaxation out of the situation as I feel I need to 'police' the situation until I feel ok.

(That's worth reading again).

Leaving the clinic, I feel relieved. It's a win to find someone who respects my back story and my skin for what it is and knows what they're doing. I plan to rebook.

Sometimes it doesn't go this way, and I've had to cut appointments short - which is always incredibly awkward. I'm old enough and experienced enough now to know when and how to speak up, but not everyone can advocate for themselves.

It took someone damaging my skin for me to decide that I was going to say my piece when it came down to saving my skin.

SKIN THEOLOGIAN'S SKINSIGHT

Twenty-eight years ago (at the time of this publication) I entered the Skin Health industry, wanting to help others achieve results that served their health and wellness. I wanted people to feel worth being cared for, supported and valued for who they are, not just what they did.

I saw for too long, the cruelty of what the corporate world could do. My Mother died prematurely, due to the stress of not being able to care for her children as a single mother while caring for herself.

It was the year that she died, from a stress-related disease, that I decided to get into a space that helped people feel good - no, feel *great* - about themselves.

A few years into the industry, I started to teach, and realized soon thereafter that my passion was supporting other Beauty Experts, Skin Professionals, Clinicians, Educators and Make-up Artists in valuing every single one of their clients not only as a good business practice, but as a human kindness and consideration for one another.

A client heard me on an expert panel and asked me which Skin Pro I would recommend her to go to -who looked like her. At that point, I realized, our industry had a long way to go. It continues to be my professional opinion that the qualifying factor of a competent Skin Pro is not their color, but rather, their empathy, expertise, track record and Cultural Intelligence.

Equity around accessible resource material for understanding skin that is Melanin-Rich was non-existent when I started. I didn't know that gap could even be filled until I realized that you don't wait for someone else to do what you have become aware of to do. I saw a gap and I wanted to fill it myself.

It started with a personal passion, then it developed into inspiring other Skin Pros within the classroom. It then progressed to creating resource materials for others to reference. And it continues now, to conferences, Beauty Institutes and Academies, Podcasts, Online courses and Webinars, Clinic training sessions and more resource materials being published.

I'm honored to continue to be a part of an evolving industry that holds space for Skin Professionals and clients of all backgrounds.

9
OFF LIMITS: MELANIN-RICH INFLAMMATORY DISEASES, DISORDERS AND TREATMENT BOUNDARIES

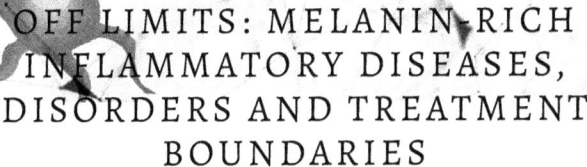

We need real, progressive change and developments ... not just talk or box-ticking...

In this chapter, you'll see:

- What the industry looks like when it comes to CQ
- The things a Pro should know
- The (potential) downsides of Dermatology

WHAT DOES THE INDUSTRY LOOK LIKE TODAY?

Today, the skincare industry showcases a promising shift towards greater inclusivity.

As covered earlier in this work and my other books, historically this industry has often overlooked the diverse needs of darker skin tones, leading to limited product options and inadequate representation in marketing and development.

However, there's been a noticeable change, with more brands recognizing the importance of catering to diverse skin tones and concerns. From expanded shade ranges in foundations and concealers to formulations addressing specific issues like hyperpigmentation, there's a growing acknowledgment of the unique requirements of melanin-rich skin.

There's an increased focus on representation, with brands actively featuring Melanin-Rich individuals in marketing campaigns and involving them in product development, signaling a move towards a more inclusive and representative skincare landscape.

While there's still progress to be made, this shift signifies a step forward in acknowledging and meeting the diverse needs of our communities.

However, there are still disparities when it comes to Dermatology, professional experience and representation. There's also the issue of whether there's still the same momentum driving these changes as there was a couple of years ago. Yes, we need to go there.

We need real, progressive change and developments in CQ - not just talk or box-ticking that doesn't get any of us anywhere.

DERMATOLOGISTS REPRESENT!

In the United States, Black dermatologists are underrepresented compared to the general population. As we mentioned earlier, only about 3%[1] of dermatologists in the U.S. identify as Black or African American, while the Black population comprises around 13% of the total population.

In the US, dermatology is classed as the second least diverse specialty in terms of the clinical workforce. From an educational perspective, one study demonstrated that 47% of dermatologists felt their training was inadequate to diagnose skin disease in skin of color. In research, race is reported in only 11% of clinical trials. A recent review of articles on cutaneous manifestations of COVID-19 revealed that studies almost exclusively featured images of patients with lighter skin.[2]

If we take these points and extrapolate them across the number of studies, resources and information available for Dermatologists then it paints a pretty poor picture of what's out there.

It's a challenge to even unpack what the percentages look like in other parts of the world as there simply isn't enough research or investigation into the levels of representation. This was a shock to me during the research for this book.

Again, it's not that only people with Melanin-Rich skin can work on or understand how to take care of Melanin-Rich skin. Not at all. But it is about representation, understanding and first-hand knowledge to break the cycle of misunderstanding and misdiagnosis.

The good news? This small percentage of individuals are working together to create resources and methods to improve the educational resources that are available, develop inclusive practices and ensure representation in textbooks and resources.

The fact of the matter is that even when you image search for most skin conditions unless you use qualifiers like race, ethnicity or terms such as "Melanin-Rich", the initial imagery you will be presented with will be these conditions or symptoms showcased on lighter skin tones. (Worth a re-read).

Again, this makes it a challenge when it comes to diagnosis, research or even just familiarizing yourself with what to look for when it comes to all shades of skin. Having to do multiple searches for every skin tone and skin condition is tiring and isn't always practical. So the likelihood is, that you go with the first image you see - and that probably isn't darker skin tones.

So, what's going on when it comes to increasing representation within Dermatology? Let's take a look at some projects and initiatives that are going on in Dermatology to try and make it easier for people to find Dermatologists, and for Dermatologists to discover more resources to give them the understanding they need.

The Black Derm Directory aims to match people looking for Dermatology professionals around the world with someone who understands their skin.

After attending IMCAS-Paris 2024, what was apparent to me was the immense visual minority that Dermatologists of Color held in comparison to all the represented Dermatologists from around the world. There were approximately 18,000 Skin Professionals in attendance at IMCAS-Paris, with a large percentage being

Dermatologists and Cosmetic Surgeons. Seeing the visual under-representation was sobering.

Vaseline has partnered with HUED (a digital health company focused on improving quality of care for Black, Latinx and Indigenous populations through education, access and data) and VisualDX (a medical informatics company that is dedicated to reducing healthcare bias by improving clinical decisions through visualization) on their See My Skin project which aims to show imagery of skin conditions on Melanin-Rich skin to educate individuals and Dermatologists.

They also provide resources on how to connect with Dermatologists and how Dermatologists can build Skin Equity into their practices. It's part of their Equitable Skincare for All Program.

Allow me to weigh in on this, as a Skin Professional, rather than an author. As a project, it seems like a great partnership - albeit there is an element of marketing and data collection to it. It should, ultimately, benefit those with Melanin-Rich skin but it's likely that this will be for commercial purposes. Business is business, but there's something about the commoditization of this much-needed imagery and resources that feels ever-so-slightly disingenuous to me.

In addition, the Skin of Color Society was established in 2004 by Susan C. Taylor, M.D. The purpose of the society is to promote awareness of and excellence within the area of special interest of dermatology — skin of color. The Society is committed to the education of healthcare providers and the general public on dermatologic health issues related to skin of color. They have membership options, resources and partnerships.

They also have a tool to help people find a Dermatologist in their area who understands Melanin-Rich skin.

In the UK in 2019/20 (the most recent stats that the health service has made available), 10% of all specialist dermatology consultations in England and Wales were with people with brown or black skin[3], but this proportion will probably vary across the country.

Based on the percentages of dermatologists in the US, it seems unlikely that these people will have seen a Dermatologist with Melanin-Rich skin, though that's not to say that those that they saw wouldn't have had adequate education. Note, I said *adequate* and not *comprehensive,* unfortunately.

Throughout the rest of Europe, there's no centralized resource or statistics on what Dermatology looks like for those with Melanin-Rich skin.

In continents where the majority of the population has Melanin-Rich skin, this representation is obviously there. Ideally, we need that knowledge and expertise in Dermatology to cross those borders and educate around the world. There's an opportunity for education, knowledge and understanding here that we should collaborate and share across the international community. CQ goes all ways, and that's important.

SKIN THEOLOGIAN'S SKINSIGHT

I've mentioned a few times, now that only 3% of Dermatologists in the US are Black, and around 4% are Hispanic[4]. Other Melanin-Rich backgrounds are even rarer in dermatology.

This leads to problems in education, recognition, diagnosis and treatment. It also starts to build a cycle where people with Melanin-Rich skin don't visit the dermatologist as they don't feel understood and decide it isn't for them. This then leads to a lack of understanding and fewer people moving into the industry because they don't get it or connect with it, and the cycle continues.

If I had to guess when it comes to Skin Pros? I would guess that the majority of professionals I meet in the US, Europe and Australia would not be considered to have Melanin-Rich skin.

Once more, I'm absolutely not saying that you need to have Melanin-Rich skin to understand it. I've met exceptionally skilled Skin Pro's who understand all shades perfectly. But it perpetuates a cycle of confusion, ignorance and clients feeling that they don't know which way to turn to get advice and care for their skin.

PRIMARY SKIN DISORDERS SKIN PROS SHOULD KNOW

Skin Pros should be aware of primary skin disorders that commonly affect Melanin-Rich skin. Here are some of the main concerns, with comprehensive definitions, characteristics, identification methods, and ways to support clients:

Post-inflammatory Hyperpigmentation (PIH)

PIH refers to darkened patches or spots that develop after inflammation or injury to the skin, commonly seen after acne, eczema, or injuries.

Characteristics: Dark brown or black patches on the skin, occurring at sites of previous inflammation or injury. They can persist for months or even years.

Identification: Identified by the presence of darker patches or spots in areas where the skin has healed from previous inflammation or injury.

Support as a Skin Pro: Provide gentle exfoliation using mild chemical exfoliants like AHAs or BHAs to aid in fading PIH. Recommend skin-brightening ingredients like vitamin C or niacinamide to even out skin tone. Emphasize sun protection as UV exposure can worsen PIH.

Keloids

Keloids are raised, thickened scars that develop due to an overgrowth of scar tissue after an injury or trauma to the skin.

Characteristics: Raised, shiny, and often larger than the original wound. They can be itchy or tender and extend beyond the borders of the original injury.

Identification: Identified by their raised, sometimes irregular appearance, extending beyond the original wound site.

Support as a Skin Pro: Advise clients to avoid unnecessary trauma to the skin, such as piercings or tattoos. Recommend silicone-based scar treatments or pressure therapy. Laser treatments and corticosteroid injections can also be beneficial under the supervision of a dermatologist.

Atrophic Scars

Atrophic scars are scarring that show up as dents or dips in the skin. It's commonly associated with conditions like acne, chickenpox, or injuries and includes boxed scars, rolled scars, and ice-pick scars.

Identification: Atrophic scars are identified by their sunken or depressed appearance on the skin, resulting from a loss of collagen and tissue.

Support as a Skin Pro: Some Skin Pros can help with multiple microneedling sessions and superficial peels. But others need to be addressed by Dermatologists. One of the more popular ways of addressing the collapsing of collagen due to extreme inflammation is a procedure that Dermatologists refer to as "Subcision". We need to know that this abnormal scarring takes place in the Dermis, and therefore for optimal results, a Dermatologist is required.

Acne Grade 3-4

Acne grades 3-4 represent a moderate to severe stage of the condition.

Identification: Can be identified by the presence of numerous inflamed papules, pustules, and possibly nodules, reflecting a moderate to severe stage of the condition with a higher degree of inflammation and skin involvement.

Support as a Skin Pro: Support for acne grades 3-4 involves implementing a comprehensive treatment plan, including targeted therapies, skincare recommendations, lifestyle education, and emotional support.

Rosacea Grade 4

Rosacea grade 4 is a severe stage of the chronic skin condition characterized by persistent facial redness and inflammation.

Identification: Pronounced facial redness, visible blood vessels, swelling, and the presence of nodules, indicative of an advanced stage of the condition with severe symptoms.

Support as a Skin Pro: Supporting those with rosacea grade 4 means implementing a tailored treatment approach - this may include prescription medications, laser therapy for vascular lesions, and offering skincare advice to alleviate symptoms and improve overall skin health.

Eczema (Dermatitis) Grade 3-4

Eczema grade 4 represents a severe stage of the inflammatory skin condition, characterized by extensive and persistent lesions, deep cracks, and potentially, widespread skin thickening.

Identification: Identifying eczema grade 4 involves recognizing the presence of extensive and chronic lesions, deep fissures, and significant skin thickening, indicating a severe and longstanding manifestation of the condition.

Support as a Skin Pro: Often eczema needs medical attention such as prescription medication and lifestyle recommendations to manage symptoms.

Suspicious lesions

Suspicious lesions refer to skin abnormalities that raise concerns about the potential for malignancy or other serious health issues, often requiring further evaluation.

Identification: Identifying suspicious lesions involves paying attention to irregularities such as changes in size, shape, color, or border of moles, lesions that bleed or itch, and asymmetry, as these may indicate a need for dermatological examination.

Support as a Skin Pro: Refer for a dermatological assessment promptly and emphasize the importance of professional evaluation with your client.

Pseudofolliculitis Barbae (Razor Bumps)

This condition occurs when shaved hair curls back into the skin, causing inflammation and bumps, commonly seen in men with curly hair patterns.

Characteristics: Inflamed, red, or dark bumps resembling acne, commonly found in areas that are shaved.

Identification: Identified by the presence of bumps or pustules in the beard area after shaving.

Support as a Skin Pro: Recommend shaving techniques that minimize irritation, such as using a single-blade razor, shaving in the direction of hair growth, and avoiding tight clothing that rubs against the skin. Provide exfoliation to prevent hair from getting trapped in the skin.

Hypopigmentation Disorders

Conditions that cause loss of skin color, such as vitiligo, where melanocytes are destroyed, leading to depigmented patches.

Characteristics: Patches of skin lighter than the surrounding area due to a lack of melanin.

Identification: Identified by the presence of depigmented patches on the skin.

Support as a Skin Pro: While repigmentation treatments require medical intervention, skin professionals can offer makeup techniques to camouflage affected areas and provide emotional support to clients. Or help them celebrate their beautiful, unique skin as is.

SKINCARE AND BEAUTY INDUSTRY

Melanin-Rich representation in the skincare industry, particularly in leadership roles and product development, historically has been limited. The same goes for education.

According to a report by McKinsey & Company[5], Black individuals held only about 3% of executive positions in the beauty industry, indicating a significant underrepresentation at the top levels.

Ensuring that Melanin-Rich representation in branding and marketing goes beyond the surface level is essential. It's too easy to have people with Melanin-Rich skin in the ads (the things that are most visible), but not to have that expertise and representation within the brand itself.

How's their calibre and extent of education around Melanin-Rich skin, for example?

Surface-level representation can feel tokenistic and insincere. Authentic representation means accurately reflecting the diversity and lived experience of the target audience, and ultimately the consumers of the products.

Meaningful representation can have a profound impact on societal perceptions and self-esteem. When individuals see themselves authentically represented in marketing and branding, it can empower them, fostering a sense of belonging and pride. It challenges stereotypes and celebrates diverse beauty standards, positively reinforcing societal attitudes.

However, research by Nielsen IQ[6] has shown that acquisitions of Black-owned and founded brands are causing consumer concern for authenticity and altered ingredients — maintaining trust while transitioning and growing should be a core principle for any brand engaging with consumers in 2024 and beyond. Engaging authentically and paying attention to the value equation will go a long way for beauty manufacturers in 2024, onward.

There's been an increasing recognition of the need for more inclusive skincare products that cater to diverse skin tones and concerns. This has led some brands to expand their ranges and include more representation in their marketing and development teams.

Here's some of the skincare brands out there that are focused on Melanin-Rich skin, or are committed to being inclusive of all skin types:

- **Bolden** focuses on addressing specific concerns of Melanin-Rich skin, offering products such as cleansers, moisturizers, and treatments designed to tackle hyperpigmentation, uneven skin tone, and dryness.
- **Black Girl Sunscreen** is dedicated to providing sun protection products formulated without harmful chemicals that often leave a white cast on darker skin tones. Their sunscreens are specifically designed to cater to the needs of black and brown skin.
- **Hyper Skin** offers products formulated to address hyperpigmentation, a common concern for people with Melanin-Rich skin. Their formulas aim to even out skin tone and reduce dark spots.
- **Nakai Skincare & Cosmetics** encourages individuals to define beauty for themselves. **Nakai** means "Be beautiful" from the Shona language of Zimbabwe.

- **456 Skin** is dedicated to providing skincare solutions specifically formulated for Melanin-Rich skin. Their products aim to address common concerns like hyperpigmentation, acne scars, and uneven skin tone, offering serums and treatments tailored to the needs of black and brown skin.

Several professional beauty brands are dedicated to promoting diversity in education within the industry. These brands prioritize inclusivity, offering resources, training, and educational initiatives that celebrate and support diversity.

- **Dermalogica PRO**. I have professionally worked with them on several projects and on an educational online training module that is FREE to all Skin Professionals. It focuses on developing confidence in treating Melanin-Rich skin.
- **Paul Mitchell Schools** are dedicated to fostering an inclusive environment for aspiring beauty professionals. They offer education and training that celebrates diversity, encouraging students to embrace and appreciate various beauty standards and cultures.

- **Sephora** has initiatives like Sephora Stands that focus on diversity and inclusion. They offer workshops and educational programs to support aspiring makeup artists and beauty enthusiasts from diverse backgrounds.

These are just a few brands that actively work toward creating educational opportunities that embrace diversity, providing platforms and resources for individuals from various backgrounds to thrive in the beauty industry.

Personally, I've also seen an increase in professionals who want to learn and brands who want to educate their teams. This is encouraging on both sides.

ACADEMIC PUBLICATIONS AND RESOURCES

Representation of Black dermatologists and researchers in academic publications has been lower compared to their counterparts.

Studies have shown disparities in publication rates and representation in scholarly journals, which can impact the diversity of research topics, perspectives, and solutions presented.

An assessment of skin of color and diversity and inclusion content of dermatologic published literature from the International Journal of Women's Dermatology showed that representation of darker skin tones in academic texts sits around 4 to 19%.[7]

The same study showed that the average percentage of overall publications relevant to Melanin-Rich skin (written as SoC, or 'Skin of Color' in the study) is quite low. The percentage of SoC articles ranged from 2.04% to 16.8% with a mean of 16.3%.

The top-performing dermatology journals in SoC were, not surprisingly, from countries with populations with SoC; however, the Journal of Cosmetic and Laser Therapy, Australasian Journal of Dermatology, and Journal of the American Academy of Dermatol Case Reports were among the top 10.

Research and higher-impact journals were among the lowest in Skin of Color rankings, including the Journal of Investigative Dermatology, Experimental Dermatology, and Journal of the American Academy of Dermatology had <5% of articles on Skin of Color.

Another study[8] found that 11% of images in Review of Dermatology were skin of color, and only two of the images were of very dark skin. Two independent teams of two reviewers classified the skin type represented in each remaining image as "non-SoC" (Fitzpatrick skin types I-IV), "SoC" (V-VI), or "indeterminate" (classification not possible).

This is pretty poor and isn't representative. It also makes appropriate representation a challenge. However, there is work going on to improve the resources and academic publications that are available all the time. I'm absolutely here for this.

The Journal of the American Academy of Dermatology have created their Skin of Color Atlas. It's a compilation of images derived from published articles in JAAD, JAAD Case Reports, and JAAD International that are meant to be used as a useful resource for the dermatology community.

The University of Michigan has this to say when it comes to looking for imagery that shows Melanin-Rich skin:

"Searching the scholarly literature on topics related to skin of color can be challenging because there are diverse ways to describe the concepts of skin color, race, and ethnicity. We encourage you to search more than one resource using multiple search terms to successfully locate relevant resources."

They then go on to list out 35(!) different search terms to use on popular online medical resources to find representative imagery. I appreciate that level of dedication, but I can't help feeling that there really must be a better way that we can come up with collectively. And believe me, I'm all about the research of vetted resources, it's what I do.

Mind the Gap is a clinical handbook of signs and symptoms and how they show on Melanin-Rich skin. The project aimed to highlight the lack of diversity in medical literature and education has become a resource to support diagnosis and education. It looks as though it's going to be developed into a community.

REAL IMPROVEMENT TO INDUSTRY INCLUSION AND DIVERSITY

The underrepresentation of people with Melanin-Rich skin in dermatology is an issue. The studies I've outlined explore barriers to entry, experiences of dermatologists in the field, and strategies to increase diversity in dermatology residency programs and academic positions. These need to be addressed, acted on and improved.

The likelihood is that there needs to be further initiatives undertaken by medical schools, professional organizations, and residency programs to recruit and support underrepresented people in dermatology. Sometimes we need to be the change we want to see or see role models that look like us to feel seen and welcome.

There are healthcare disparities throughout dermatology, focusing on access to care, misdiagnosis, and different treatment outcomes for patients with Melanin-Rich skin. There is progress when it comes to advocating for more equitable healthcare practices, but it's slower than it could be.

Outreach and educational programs aimed at attracting and mentoring underrepresented people into becoming Skin Pros (in whatever capacity that may be). These programs often focus on mentorship, educational support, and exposure to the field. I'm seeing more and more of this happening and frankly, it couldn't come together soon enough.

MEDI-AESTHETIC COLLABORATIONS SERVE MELANIN-RICH CLIENTS

As I mentioned earlier, the bridge between Dermatologists and Skin Professionals is pivotal in fostering holistic skin health. We must understand their roles as allies, contributing to comprehensive skin care.

Dermatologists, with their specialized medical training, offer expertise in diagnosing and treating higher grades of inflammatory diseases and disorders. In such cases, their intervention becomes indispensable, ensuring accurate diagnosis and management.

While dermatologists excel in addressing complex conditions like severe acne, eczema, or psoriasis, Skin Professionals provide invaluable support in preventive care, maintenance, and overall skin wellness.

They specialize in personalized routines, offering guidance on daily care, tailored treatments, and lifestyle adjustments to enhance skin health.

There are instances where seeing a dermatologist exclusively might be necessary, especially in cases requiring systemic, medical intervention, prescription medications, or advanced treatments beyond the scope of Skin Pros.

Embracing this collaborative approach means that our mutual clients receive comprehensive care - this is especially important when it comes to Melanin-Rich skin that doesn't always benefit from this collaborative approach. By building these networks and resources, it becomes easier to work together and get the best results.

SKIN THEOLOGIAN'S SKINSIGHT

Dermatologists have the training and expertise to accurately diagnose and manage higher-grade skin conditions. They can differentiate between various skin disorders that may appear similar, ensuring an accurate diagnosis. Additionally, they can prescribe medications, including systemic treatments like oral medications or biologics, that require medical oversight and monitoring.

Certain conditions, especially severe Acne or Psoriasis, may need advanced procedures that are best handled by a medical professional.

When a client with severe Acne, for instance, undergoing a treatment like Accutane (Isotretinoin), seeks support from a Skin Professional, there are specific ways the Skin Professional can assist while the client continues under the care of a dermatologist.

This could be through complementary skincare, monitoring and guidance or lifestyle recommendations. I.e.:

- Deeply hydrating the skin
- Soothing and sedating the skin
- Omitting all exfoliating actives, like AHA's, BHA and Retinoids
- Restoring the skin's barrier function

Please also note that as Skin Pros, we need to know the duration of time that is required to not re-introduce these actives, after having completed a Dermatologist prescribed treatment, like Isotretinoin. After which, it is recommended to wait 10-12 months from their last dose before the use of Hydroxy Acids or Renewing Actives.

In essence, while certain skin conditions require the expertise of a dermatologist, Skin Pros play a pivotal role in supporting clients with their skin health recovery.

This isn't just exclusive to Melanin-Rich skin, but understanding the pathways and process becomes even more important when you're dealing with clients who may not feel represented or may have been let down in the past.

THE 3-TIP PROFESSIONAL GUIDE TO CLIENT CARE

When it comes to client care, professionalism and expertise is essential. But so is treating every client who enters your space as their own person. This is a key part of CQ, but is also a key part of a people-focused approach, and customer service.

Let's get into it. The 3-tip guide for client care.

LEAD WITH HUMANITY

Now that we have covered the appropriateness and partnership of Dermatology care, let's talk about when clients are back in our care after any specified duration of treatment has concluded.

There are still cautions that we need to bear in mind when it comes to Melanin-Rich skin. Remember, with darker skin, especially higher levels of Acne, there are greater levels of hidden erythema. So, supportive professional approaches, by sitting down with a client are critical to our CQ interaction with clients.

Here are the 3-Tips, along with a few examples that I have shared in many training sessions with other Skin Professionals:

> **Tip #1: Always Lead with Humanity. Be Empathetic. Treat The Client in the skin FIRST. Not the Other Way Around.**
> **Tip #2: Lead with What You Can Do, Not What You Cannot Do.**
> **Tip #3: Lead with What is Great About Their Skin, Not What is Wrong With Their Skin**

Example 1: Client with Melanin-Rich skin who has Grade 4 Acne and wants Microneedling.

Tip #1: Listen and acknowledge the concerns and challenges that the client with Acne has expressed. Refer to the client first, never the Acne. Remember, we treat the person in the skin, not the other way around. Clients will feel a human connection from you, and not feel dehumanized or disconnected.

Tip #2: Share the supportive options that you can offer the client today, while they're with you, like a possible scalp or MLD body massage. Explain the benefits of relaxation where Acne is concerned, due to higher cortisol levels. Reducing stress can greatly de-escalate inflammatory mediators within the body, improving stress-related exacerbated Acne conditions.

Secondly, share and inform the client why Microneedling would not support their skin health with their current stage of Acne. It could lead to more inflammation, resulting in greater levels of PIH. The inflammation at this stage is within the Dermal layer, and this is best addressed by a dermatologist. You are here to support, once the dermatologist's directives have been able to control the deeper inflammation.

Tip #3: Ask the client or acknowledge for the client what is great about their skin. I cannot stress the value of this enough. Most clients are anticipating a feeling of shame about their skin concerns. As Skin Professionals, we can change that narrative. And show them that we understand that they are BIGGER than their skin concern. You SEE them. You HEAR them. You ACKNOWLEDGE what is great about their skin. And our Goal is to support that more while addressing the other concerns simultaneously.

*This is one suggested example, but try to work through the following scenarios or any others you may have in your space and see how much deeper rapport is established. Go ahead, I dare you.

Example 2: A Client with Melanin-Rich skin wants a Peel percentage that you feel they are not suited for.

Tip #1: How Can You Lead With Humanity?

_____

_____

_____

_____

Tip #2: Lead With What You Can Do vs. What You Cannot Do. How Could This Look?

_____

_____

_____

_____

Tip #3: Lead With What Is Great About Their Skin. What Could You Highlight Here?

_____

_____

_____

_____

Do this exercise as a team or for yourself with the following: conditions with clients with Melanin-Rich skin.

- Client With Eczema
- Client with Dermal Hyperpigmentation
- Client who wants to get an Ablative Laser treatment done with your C02 laser she saw.
- Client who overprocesses their skin with aggressive treatments.
- Client with Rosacea (Grade 1)

I hope you see that the opportunities for fostering deeper bonds are only growing with more and more practical applications of this 3-Tip Pro approach, whenever a client has a concern.

Leading with humanity as a Skin Pro means taking a client-centric approach.

This client-centric approach fosters a deeper connection, empathy, and understanding, ensuring that the client feels seen, heard, and valued beyond the surface of their skin. Ultimately, leading with humanity in skincare takes it further than "just" treatments, creating a compassionate and inclusive space that honors each client's unique story and journey toward skin wellness.

CONCLUSION

There are so many factors to take into consideration when you're working with a client and taking care of their skin. That doesn't change.

However, there is a knowledge and skills gap when it comes to working with clients with Melanin-Rich skin. They might have needs that are individual to them, but that is absolutely the same with every single client.

What we need is more knowledge, growth, experience, connection and confidence in working with every single type of skin. Not just the type we see the most often, or the type that resembles our own the most.

There are so many opportunities for our industry to do better, and thankfully we are moving more and more towards that. I thank you for that as a committed professional who understands the brilliance of Skin Health Equity.

GLOSSARY OF RESOURCES AND TERMS

It takes a village to effect change. This glossary aims to unlock knowledge about Melanin-Rich skin, diving deep into the terminology that defines and underpins everything you need to know about skincare.

Whether you use it as a reference point, or take it to understand what's going on with your clients, this Melanin-Rich skin glossary is your companion on a fascinating journey through melanin and its impact on our skin.

MELANIN-RICH GLOSSARY

Melanin-Rich Online Courses

Dermalogica Pro
(FREE Course)Treating Melanin Rich Skin
(Available in 7 languages)
www.treatingmelaninrichskin.com

Academies Catering To Underrepresented Education

The Skin Barrier Academy
Nichelle Mosley
QUEEN CITY BEAUTY GROUP + WELLNESS
SKIN BARRIER ACADEMY
WWW.QUEENCITYBEAUTYGROUP.COM
WWW.SKINBARRIERACADEMY.COM

Institute of Beauty Aesthetics, PC DBA: School of Beauty Aesthetic Institute
Latoya Beverly, CLT, LSO, LEHP
www.schoolofbeautyaestheticsinstitute.org

Champion's Beauty Institute School Of Esthetics
Portland's 1st Multicultural Esthetics Program
Amantha Hood
Director
www.cbi.life/esthetics

Authors and Other Works

Dija Ayodele
(Book) BLACK SKIN
@dijaayodele
(Fee Paying Online Courses) https://www.blackskindirectory.com/

JoElle Lee
Skin Of Color Expert and Author
(Book) Multi-Cutural Skin Treatments
(Fee Paying Online Courses) https://www.joellelee.com/online-courses

Fearless Beauties
(Book) Fearless Beauties 3rd Edition
(Online Certification)
https://www.fearlessbeauties.org/fbevents
https://www.fearlessbeauties.org/

The Skin Testaments: 10 Tips to Grow Confidently in Your Skin
Candis White (Cozi)
Author | Instructor | Lead Esthetician
https://theskintestaments.com/

Inclusion Experts

Sam Marshall
Trans and Non-Binary Expert
https://www.betransaware.co.uk/
https://ght.org.uk/

Organizations for Professionals

Skin Of Color Society
https://www.skinofcolorsociety.org/
IG:@skinofcolorsociety

Pema
Professional Esthetician Membership Association
IG: @pemacanada
https://www.pemacanada.com/

The British Beauty Council's DEI Committee
https://britishbeautycouncil.com/dei-committee/
IG: @britishbeautycouncil

British Association of Beauty Therapy and Cosmetology [BABTAC]
https://www.babtac.com/
IG: @babtac

City & Guilds Council - UK
https://cityandguildsfoundation.org/about-us/our-impact/#impact-report

Terms

Copper
A mineral that plays a role in the production of melanin within melanocytes, contributing to skin pigmentation.

Dendrite Arm
A branch-like extension from a dendritic cell or melanocyte, aiding in cellular communication and pigment distribution.

Dendritic Cell
A specialized immune cell involved in the skin's defense mechanisms, interacting with melanocytes and supporting immune responses.

Dermis
The layer of skin beneath the epidermis contains connective tissue, blood vessels, and nerve endings.

Epidermal/Dermal Junction (DEJ)
The interface between the epidermis and dermis is crucial for skin strength and elasticity.

Epidermis
The outer layer of the skin responsible for protecting the body from the environment.

Eumelanin
A type of melanin pigment less soluble in skin cells, often related to darker skin tones and influencing the time it takes to treat hyperpigmentation in Melanin-Rich skin.

Hypodermis
The deepest layer of the skin, composed of fat and connective tissue, provides insulation and cushioning.

Hypopigmentation
A condition characterized by areas of skin becoming lighter due to reduced melanin production or loss of pigment cells.

Hyperpigmentation
Darkening of the skin caused by an overproduction of melanin, resulting in patches or spots that are darker than the surrounding skin.

Keratinocyte or Corneocyte Cell
Skin cells found in the epidermis, responsible for producing keratin, forming the skin's protective barrier.

Lentigines
Commonly known as age spots or UV damage spots, these are localized areas of increased pigmentation on the skin.

Melanin
A pigment produced by melanocytes that determines skin, hair, and eye color and provides protection against UV radiation.

Melanin-Rich
Melanin-Rich refers to and celebrates skin with a higher concentration of the pigment melanin. It's a term that's used to describe a client's skin.

Melanocyte Cell
Specialized cells in the skin, are responsible for producing and distributing melanin.

Melanocyte Receptors
Structures on melanocytes that receive signals, influencing melanin production in response to various stimuli.

Melanogenesis
The process of melanin production within melanocytes.

Melanosome
An organelle within melanocytes where melanin pigment is synthesized and stored.

Melanotic Disorder
Also known as Pigmentary Disorder, involves Genetic implications on the Melanocyte Cell.

Melasma/Chloasma (Pregnancy Mask)
A skin condition characterized by patches of hyperpigmentation, often occurring during pregnancy or due to hormonal changes.

Pheomelanin
A type of melanin pigment is more soluble in skin cells, potentially making hyperpigmentation easier to treat compared to eumelanin-dominant skin.

Pendulous Melanocyte
A damaged melanocyte tilted on its axis, with a dendrite pointing into the dermis, possibly contributing to pigmentary disorders.

Post Inflammatory Hyperpigmentation (PIH)
Darkened areas of the skin that occur after inflammation or injury, often resolving over time.

Tyrosinase
An enzyme crucial for melanin synthesis within melanocytes.

Tyrosinase Cascade
A series or chain of complex processes within the Melanin synthesis stage.

Tyrosine
An amino acid involved in melanin production, serving as a precursor for melanogenesis.

Key Ingredients and Benefits for Melanin-Rich Skin

Hydroxy Acids
Chemical exfoliants such as Alpha and Beta Hydroxy Acids help even skin tone, promote cell turnover and reduce hyperpigmentation in melanin-rich skin.

Tyrosinase Inhibitors
Compounds that inhibit the enzyme tyrosinase, involved in melanin production, thereby reducing dark spots and hyperpigmentation in individuals with melanin-rich skin.

Hydroquinone
A Skin-Lightening Agent that inhibits melanin production, effectively treating hyperpigmentation issues in melanin-rich skin.

Retinol
Vitamin A derivatives stimulate collagen production, promote skin renewal, and help fade dark spots and hyperpigmentation in all skin.

Niacinamide (Vitamin B3)
Known for its anti-inflammatory and skin-brightening properties, Niacinamide helps improve uneven skin tone and reduce hyperpigmentation.

Vitamin C (Ascorbic Acid)
A powerful antioxidant that helps to inhibit melanin production, lighten dark spots, and protect the skin from environmental damage.

Licorice Extract
Contains compounds that may help lighten dark spots and hyperpigmentation while soothing the skin.

Kojic Acid
A natural Skin-Lightening Agent derived from mushrooms that can help reduce hyperpigmentation and even out skin tone.

Alpha Arbutin
An extract that inhibits melanin production and is often used for its skin-brightening effects.

Glycolic Acid
A type of Alpha Hydroxy Acid (AHA) that exfoliates the skin, helps with cell turnover, and can improve the appearance of dark spots.

Azelaic Acid
Treats hyperpigmentation and inflammatory skin conditions, promoting an even skin tone.

Modalities/Equipment Procedures

Laser
A device that emits intense, focused light of a specific wavelength, used for various medical and cosmetic applications.

Ablative Laser
A laser that removes layers of skin by vaporization, often employed for skin resurfacing.

Non-Ablative Laser
A laser that stimulates collagen production without removing the outer skin layer, commonly used for skin rejuvenation.

Wavelengths
Specific ranges of electromagnetic radiation emitted by lasers influence their interaction with tissues.

Chromophores
Target molecules in tissues that absorb specific wavelengths of light during laser treatments.

Selective PhotoThermolysis
The principle of selectively targeting specific tissues using lasers based on their absorption characteristics.

Superficial Peels
Cosmetic treatments involve the application of mild acids to exfoliate the outer layer of the skin.

Microdermabrasion
A non-invasive exfoliation technique that removes the outermost layer of skin using microcrystals or a diamond-tipped wand.

Microneedling
A procedure involving the use of tiny needles to create controlled micro-injuries, promoting collagen and elastin production.

HydraFacials
A non-invasive facial treatment that combines cleansing, exfoliation, extraction, hydration, and antioxidant protection.

Subcision
A surgical technique used to treat depressed scars by releasing fibrous bands underneath the skin's surface.

Dermabrasion
A surgical procedure that mechanically removes the outer layers of skin, commonly used for scar revision or skin resurfacing.

NOTES

INTRODUCTION

1. Improving skin tone evaluation in machine learning, Google https://skintone.google/
2. Beauty's next big opportunity: Melanin-Rich skincare, Vogue Business https://www.voguebusiness.com/beauty/beautys-next-big-opportunity-melanin-rich-skincare
3. What Is 'Melanin Safe' Skincare — & Is It Really Necessary?, Refinery29, https://www.refinery29.com/en-us/melanin-safe-skincare
4. Major retailers bring $14 billion in revenue to Black-owned brands, CNBC - https://www.cnbc.com/2023/08/11/black-owned-brands-get-boost-from-retailers-like-nordstrom-macys.html#:~:text=%2414%20billion%20in%20revenue%20has,nonprofit%20organization%20Fifteen%20Percent%20Pledge.
5. Meeting the needs of black consumers in 2023, NielsenIQ - https://nielseniq.com/global/en/insights/analysis/2023/meeting-the-needs-of-black-beauty-consumers-in-2023/#:~:text=As%20a%20group%2C%20Black%20Americans,the%20total%20market's%209%25%20growth.
6. Black beauty brands and consumers: Where do we go from here?, McKinsey, https://www.mckinsey.com/industries/retail/our-insights/black-beauty-brands-and-consumers-where-do-we-go-from-here
7. Black representation in the beauty industry, McKinsey - https://www.mckinsey.com/industries/consumer-packaged-goods/our-insights/black-representation-in-the-beauty-industry

1. MELANIN-RICH: A GLOBAL EMBRACE

1. Global Melanin Rich searches in 5 year period, Google Trends
https://trends.google.com/trends/explore?date=today%205-y&q=melanin%20rich&hl=en-GB
2. #melaninrich, Instagram https://www.instagram.com/explore/tags/melaninrich
3. #melaninrich, TikTok
https://www.tiktok.com/tag/melaninrich

2. THE GRACE & TRUTH OF SKIN HEALTH EQUITY

1. Skin color in dermatology textbooks: An updated evaluation and analysis, British Journal of Dermatology
https://www.jaad.org/article/S0190-9622(20)30700-3/pdf
2. Why Melanin-Rich skin care lines are beauty's most necessary launches, Cosmetics Business
https://cosmeticsbusiness.com/news/article_page/Why_melanin-rich_skin_care_lines_are_beautys_most_necessary_launches/207718

4. MELANOCYTES: THE GOOD | THE BAD | THE SCIENCE

1. The Antimicrobial Properties of Melanocytes, Melanosomes and Melanin
and the Evolution of Black Skin, https://www.sciencedirect.com/science/article/abs/pii/S0022519301923318
2. Skin of Color Skin Care Needs: Results of a Multi-Center-Based Survey, https://jddonline.com/articles/skin-of-color-skin-care-

needs-results-of-a-multi-center-based-survey-S1545961622P0709X/
3. Effects of Topical Retinoids on Acne and Post-inflammatory Hyperpigmentation in Patients with Skin of Color: A Clinical Review and Implications for Practice, Therapy in Practice, https://link.springer.com/article/10.1007/s40257-021-00643-2
4. The Antimicrobial Properties of Melanocytes, Melanosomes and Melanin and the Evolution of Black Skin, Journey of Theoretical Biology, https://www.sciencedirect.com/science/article/abs/pii/S0022519301923318
5. Black patients and skin cancer, American Academy of Dermatology
    https://www.aamc.org/news/why-are-so-many-black-patients-dying-skin-cancer#:~:text=Understanding%20the%20risks&text=Black%20people%20are%20far%20less,provides%20from%20damaging%20ultraviolet%20rays.

5. STEP INTO THE (MELANIN-RICH) CLASSROOM

1. Decolonizing global health: what should be the target of this movement and where does it lead us?, Global Health Research and Policy https://ghrp.biomedcentral.com/articles/10.1186/s41256-022-00237-3
2. Inclusive Skin Color Project, UCSF Library, https://guides.ucsf.edu/c.php?g=1081119&p=9159811
3. Improving Representation of Skin of Color in a Medical School Preclerkship Dermatology Curriculum, Springer, https://link.springer.com/article/10.1007/s40670-021-01473-x
4. Effects of Topical Retinoids on Acne and Post-inflammatory Hyperpigmentation in Patients with Skin of Color: A Clinical Review and Implications for Practice, Therapy in Practice, https://link.springer.com/article/10.1007/s40257-021-00643-2
5. The Antimicrobial Properties of Melanocytes, Melanosomes and Melanin and the Evolution of Black Skin, Journal of Theoretical

Biology, https://www.sciencedirect.com/science/article/abs/pii/ S0022519301923318?via%3Dihub

7. LET'S GET CLINICAL

1. The Antimicrobial Properties of Melanocytes, Melanosomes and Melanin and the Evolution of Black Skin, Journal of Theoretical Biology, https://www.sciencedirect.com/science/article/abs/pii/ S0022519301923318
2. A review of genetic disorders of hypopigmentation: lessons learned from the biology of melanocytes, Expert Dermatology, https://pubmed.ncbi.nlm.nih.gov/19555431/
3. Diversity, Equity and Inclusion in the Beauty Sector, MBS Intelligence, https://cewuk.co.uk/wp-content/uploads/2022/02/DEI-IN-THE-BEAUTY-SECTOR.pdf
4. Hyperpigmentation: types, diagnostics and targeted treatment options, , https://onlinelibrary.wiley.com/doi/pdf/10.1111/jdv.12048

9. OFF LIMITS: MELANIN-RICH INFLAMMATORY DISEASES, DISORDERS AND TREATMENT BOUNDARIES

1. Embracing diversity in dermatology: Creation of a culture of equity and inclusion in dermatology, International Journal of Women's Dermatology https://www.ncbi.nlm.nih.gov/pmc/articles/PMC8484952/
2. Dermatology is finally talking about race, British Journal of Dermatology
   https://onlinelibrary.wiley.com/doi/full/10.1111/bjd.20599
3. Ensuring equity of access to care when redesigning dermatology pathways, NHS England

https://www.england.nhs.uk/long-read/ensuring-equity-of-access-to-care-when-redesigning-dermatology-pathways/

4. Racial disparities in dermatology, Archives of dermatological research
https://jamanetwork.com/journals/jamadermatology/article-abstract/2618147

5. Black Representation in the Beauty Industry, McKinsey https://www.mckinsey.com/industries/consumer-packaged-goods/our-insights/black-representation-in-the-beauty-industry

6. Meeting the needs of black beauty consumers in 2023, Nielsen IQ
https://nielseniq.com/global/en/insights/analysis/2023/meeting-the-needs-of-black-beauty-consumers-in-2023

7. Assessment of skin of color and diversity and inclusion content of dermatologic published literature: An analysis and call to action, International Journal of Women's Dermatology
https://www.sciencedirect.com/science/article/pii/S2352647521000538#bib0002

8. Assessment of skin of color and diversity and inclusion content of dermatologic published literature: An analysis and call to action, Journal of the American Academy of Dermatology
https://www.jaad.org/article/S0190-9622(22)00521-7/fulltext

www.ingramcontent.com/pod-product-compliance
Lightning Source LLC
Chambersburg PA
CBHW051539020426
42333CB00016B/2003